T0296884

Endoscopic Atlas of Pediatric Otolaryngology

Jeffrey Cheng · John P. Bent

Editors

Endoscopic Atlas of Pediatric Otolaryngology

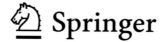

Editors
Jeffrey Cheng, M.D., F.A.A.P.
Division of Pediatric Otolaryngology
Cohen Children's Medical Center
Assistant Professor of Otolaryngology
  – Head and Neck Surgery
Hofstra North Shore – LIJ School
  of Medicine
New Hyde Park, NY, USA

John P. Bent, M.D.
Professor of Otorhinolaryngology
  – Head and Neck Surgery
Department of Otorhinolaryngology
Montefiore Medical Center
Medical Arts Pavilion
Bronx, NY, USA

ISBN 978-3-319-29469-8   ISBN 978-3-319-29471-1   (eBook)
DOI 10.1007/978-3-319-29471-1

Library of Congress Control Number: 2016937406

© Springer International Publishing Switzerland 2016
This work is subject to copyright. All rights are reserved by the Publisher, whether the whole or part of the material is concerned, specifically the rights of translation, reprinting, reuse of illustrations, recitation, broadcasting, reproduction on microfilms or in any other physical way, and transmission or information storage and retrieval, electronic adaptation, computer software, or by similar or dissimilar methodology now known or hereafter developed.
The use of general descriptive names, registered names, trademarks, service marks, etc. in this publication does not imply, even in the absence of a specific statement, that such names are exempt from the relevant protective laws and regulations and therefore free for general use.
The publisher, the authors and the editors are safe to assume that the advice and information in this book are believed to be true and accurate at the date of publication. Neither the publisher nor the authors or the editors give a warranty, express or implied, with respect to the material contained herein or for any errors or omissions that may have been made.

Printed on acid-free paper

This Springer imprint is published by Springer Nature
The registered company is Springer International Publishing AG Switzerland

Preface

The idea for this book came about from two different perspectives. First, not a day in the office goes by without a parent or caregiver asking me for more anatomic detail about their child's condition. Lacking natural artistic and drawing abilities, I have found that showing the families a picture of the pathology and/or anatomy is extremely valuable in our discussions and joint decision-making process. Secondly, optical endoscopy has revolutionized imaging in the head and neck. It has allowed illumination, magnification, and visualization in spaces that are not fully appreciated with the naked eye. Endoscopes offer some advantages even beyond binocular microscopy, including an increased field of view and lack of line-of-sight limitations. This allows us to look around the corners, with improved brightness and clarity.

This atlas is by no means meant to be a comprehensive review of pediatric otolaryngology disorders but rather to provide some illustrative images, along with a brief discussion of clinical considerations, and to help educate our patients, families, caregivers, medical students, residents, fellows, and other allied health professionals. Most, but not all, of the images were captured with an optical endoscope. This is meant to stimulate thought processes in the future for further possibilities for capturing images, as other types of image-capturing technologies grow and expand with time. The content is divided by anatomic area in the head and neck: ear, nose, throat/mouth, and airway/aerodigestive tract. We feel that this will be a helpful resource for not just the otolaryngologist who cares for children but the far more numerous pediatricians and other caregivers, such as speech and language pathologists, nurses, physician assistants, medical assistants, nurse practitioners, and audiologists. Our hope is that this is just the beginning of an imaging collection, and that there will be continued discovery and contribution to further improve this atlas.

New Hyde Park, NY, USA   Jeffrey Cheng
Bronx, NY, USA   John P. Bent

Acknowledgements

For all of my mentors, teachers, and colleagues who have inspired me, thank you. And a special note of appreciation to my patients and families, as they are our greatest teachers.

Jeffrey Cheng

I credit Jeff for his leadership, initiative, and vision to make this important text a reality. It immediately appeals as an educational reference for families and other providers, but its greatest role will be to serve as both a template and a trailblazer for future enhancements.

John P. Bent

Contents

Contributors

Jeffrey Cheng, M.D., F.A.A.P Division of Pediatric Otolaryngology, Cohen Children's Medical Center, Assistant Professor of Otolaryngology – Head and Neck Surgery, Hofstra North Shore – LIJ School of Medicine, New Hyde Park, NY, USA

Nathan Gonik, M.D., M.H.S.A. Department of Otolaryngology, Wayne State University School of Medicine, Children's Hospital of Michigan, Detroit, MI, USA

Bianca Siegel, M.D. Ear, Nose, and Throat Services (Otolaryngology), Wayne State University School of Medicine, Children's Hospital of Michigan, Detroit, MI, USA

Lee P. Smith, M.D. Division of Pediatric Otolaryngology, Cohen Children's Medical Center, Otolaryngology — Head and Neck Surgery, Hofstra Northwell School of Medicine, New Hyde Park, NY, USA

Elena B. Willis Woodson, M.D. Otolaryngology and Audiology, Oklahoma University, Oklahoma City, OK, USA

External and Middle Ear

Bianca Siegel

External Ear

The external ear consists of the auricle and the external auditory canal and functions to allow sound in to reach and vibrate the tympanic membrane. The auricle forms embryologically from the hillocks of His, and any interruption or abnormality in this process can result in congenital abnormality of the auricle. The external auditory canal forms from the first pharyngeal cleft, and abnormalities in this development can result in auditory canal stenosis or atresia. These congenital anomalies are typically evident at the time of birth and are often associated with other congenital anomalies and syndromes [1].

Examination of the external ear should focus on the auricle and ear canal. Auricles should be examined for symmetry and evaluated for any anatomic abnormality, such as microtia, prominauris, or preauricular pit. Additionally, the presence of proptosis or any asymmetry between the two ears should be noted. Although an important part of the physical examination, examination of the auricle is beyond the scope of this text. Examination of the external auditory canal should evaluate the patency of the canal as well as the presence of any significant cerumen or foreign material within the ear canal, and endoscopy can be quite helpful in examining the ear canal. Any masses or lesions of the ear canal should be noted, as should the presence of drainage or dermatologic conditions involving the skin of the ear canal. Any lesions or abnormalities in the external ear can contribute to hearing loss, which is an important clinical consideration.

External Ear Canal

Normal Anatomy

The ear canal runs from the outer ear to the middle ear in an anterior-inferior direction. The lateral third of the ear canal is cartilaginous and the medial two-thirds are bony. Cerumen is a normal finding in the ear canal and contributes to cleaning and lubrication of the ear canal. Figure 1.1 shows a normal external ear canal.

Cerumen Impaction

Excess cerumen in the ear canal can result in cerumen impaction (Fig. 1.2). This can result in discomfort and conductive hearing loss, and it prevents adequate visualization of the tympanic membrane. Treatment options may include cerumenolytic solutions and manual removal of the cerumen.

B. Siegel, M.D. (✉)
Ear, Nose, and Throat Services (Otolaryngology),
Wayne State University School of Medicine,
Children's Hospital of Michigan, Detroit, MI, USA
e-mail: siegel.bianca@gmail.com

© Springer International Publishing Switzerland 2016
J. Cheng, J.P. Bent (eds.), *Endoscopic Atlas of Pediatric Otolaryngology*,
DOI 10.1007/978-3-319-29471-1_1

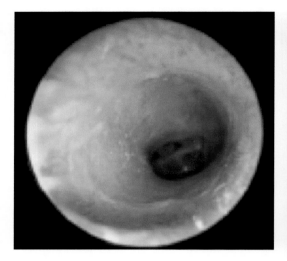

Fig. 1.1 Normal ear canal—right ear

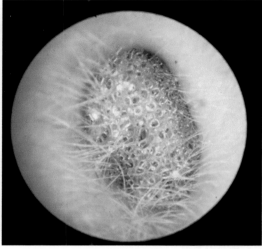

Fig. 1.3 Sponge in ear canal (reprinted from the Hawke Library [hawkelibrary.com]; with permission)

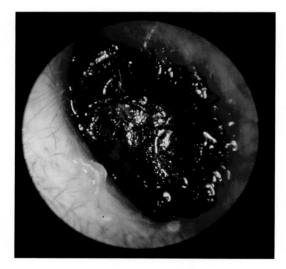

Fig. 1.2 Impacted cerumen (reprinted from the Hawke Library [hawkelibrary.com]; with permission)

Foreign Body

Foreign bodies in the ear are common in the pediatric population. Common foreign bodies include organic materials, such as plants, and other vegetable matter or insects, and inorganic materials, such as plastic pieces, beads, and sponges (Fig. 1.3) [2]. Removal can typically be performed in the office using irrigation/suctioning methods or mechanical extraction using forceps and other instruments [3]. Following complete removal of the foreign body, it is important to examine the ear canal for any abrasions as well as thoroughly examine the tympanic membrane.

Otitis Externa

Otitis externa, also commonly called "swimmer's ear," refers to diffuse inflammation of the skin of the ear canal, which can also extend to involve other structures, such as the tympanic membrane or the pinna [4]. Often, there is a significant amount of debris in the inflamed ear canal and significant edema of the ear canal is another common finding (Fig. 1.4). Acute otitis externa is most commonly caused by bacterial pathogens such as *Pseudomonas aeruginosa* and *Staphylococcus aureus* and occurs commonly in swimmers, although predisposing factors such as humidity, local trauma, and ear canal obstruction have also been implicated [5]. Acute otitis externa typically presents with otalgia and aural fullness; physical examination findings include tenderness of the tragus, ear canal edema, and otorrhea. It is important to rule out other diagnoses, such as retained foreign body or otomycosis, which may present similarly; these can typically be ruled out by a thorough physical examination.

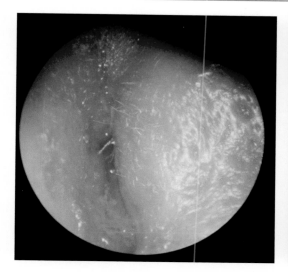

Fig. 1.4 Severe acute otitis externa with ear canal edema (reprinted from the Hawke Library [hawkelibrary.com]; with permission)

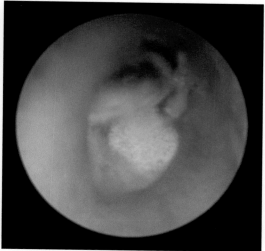

Fig. 1.5 Otomycosis—left ear

Otomycosis

Otomycosis is a superficial fungal infection of the external ear canal that typically presents with otalgia and pruritus. Physical examination findings can be very similar to otitis externa; therefore, a high index of suspicion is important in making the correct diagnosis, particularly in patients who have not responded to treatment for bacterial otitis externa. Findings often include tenderness of the ear canal and purulent drainage; however, the finding of visible white fungal elements is pathognomonic for otomycosis (Fig. 1.5) [4]. The most commonly implicated pathogens are *Candida* and *Aspergillus* species [6]. Predisposing factors include a humid climate, presence of cerumen, frequent use of antibiotic or steroid ototopical medications, and local trauma [7].

Osteoma

Osteomas of the external auditory canal are rare benign neoplasms that are usually found incidentally, as symptoms are rare unless they are completely obstructive. Lesions are typically unilateral and solitary, and there are no known causative factors [8]. Physical examination typi-

cally reveals a partially obstructed ear canal, and the diagnosis is confirmed by radiographic imaging (Fig. 1.6).

Exostoses

Exostoses of the external auditory canal are bony growths that are a distinct entity from osteomas, occurring almost exclusively in surfers. Unlike osteomas, exostoses are typically bilateral and multiple (Fig. 1.7), and they are also typically asymptomatic unless they become large enough to become obstructive. Surgical intervention is the mainstay of treatment for symptomatic exostoses [9]. Exostoses are thought to represent a reactive condition secondary to recurrent cold water immersions, and ears with exostoses are commonly referred to as "surfer's ears." Preventive measures, including the use of earplugs and wet suit hoods, have been shown to help prevent the onset of exostoses [10].

Inflammatory Polyp

Polypoid tissue in the ear canal can be seen for a variety of reasons and is typically inflammatory in nature (Fig. 1.8). Underlying causes must be

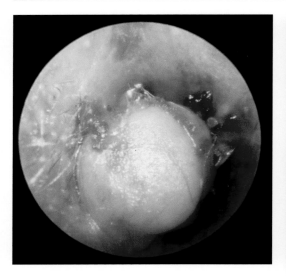

Fig. 1.6 Osteoma of external ear canal—right ear (reprinted from the Hawke Library [hawkelibrary.com]; with permission)

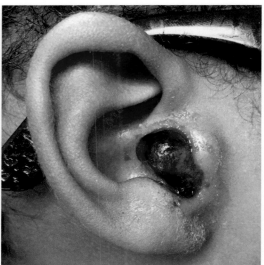

Fig. 1.8 Polyp in external ear canal

described presenting as a mass within the ear canal and should remain in the differential diagnosis [12].

Tympanic Membrane and Middle Ear

The tympanic membrane acts as an integral component in addition to the ossicular chain—malleus, incus, and stapes—in the impedance-matching function for transducing sound waves from an air medium into the fluid-conducting medium within the inner ear and membranous labyrinth [13, 14]. In addition to an intact, mobile tympanic membrane and ossicular chain for normal hearing, the middle ear cavity must be able to maintain ventilation as an air-containing space. Maturity and function of the Eustachian tube are integral in this function and physiology. Much of the tympanic membrane and middle ear pathology that affects the pediatric population is centered on Eustachian tube physiology.

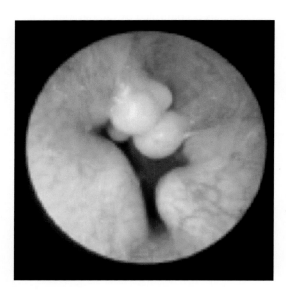

Fig. 1.7 Exostoses of external ear canal

considered. In the pediatric population, polypoid tissue can be secondary to a foreign body in the ear canal or an extruding tympanostomy tube or be secondary to other processes. Cholesteatoma is the most common underlying condition; however, other underlying benign and malignant neoplasms must also be considered [11]. Rhabdomyosarcoma is an exceedingly rare diagnosis, but it has been

Normal Anatomy

The normal structure of the tympanic membrane consists of three histologic layers, including a lateral squamous epithelial, middle fibrous, and medial endothelial/mucosal layer [15]. A normal tympanic membrane with well-ventilated middle right and left ear can be found in Fig. 1.9. There are also two primary areas of the tympanic membrane, which include the pars tensa and pars flaccida [15]. The pars tensa composes most of the tympanic membrane and is the stronger of the two areas, with the pars flaccida subject to greater Eustachian tube dysfunction processes [16].

Pressure Equalization Tube (PET) or Tympanostomy Tube

Tympanostomy tube placement is one of the most commonly performed pediatric surgical procedures in the USA; the most common indications are chronic otitis media with effusion and recurrent acute otitis media [17]. Figure 1.10 shows a tympanostomy tube in place. Patients can develop a foreign body reaction to tympanostomy tubes, which presents with granulation tissue in and around the tube. A tympanostomy tube granuloma is shown in Fig. 1.11. Tympanostomy tubes come in a variety of shapes and sizes, although the most common type is shaped like a grommet. Patients who require more long-term ventilation tubes may have a

"t-tube," which is a longer lasting type of tube. A variety of materials are used to construct the tube, but the most commonly used materials are plastics such as silicone and Teflon or metals such as titanium or stainless steel.

Tympanosclerosis

Prior inflammatory, infectious, or iatrogenic (e.g., tympanostomy tube insertion or trauma) insults may result in fibrosis and scarring of the middle fibrous layer of the tympanic membrane. In general, this is of relatively little clinical consequence; however, it should be noted on otoscopic examination, as seen in Fig. 1.12.

Bullous Myringitis

Bullous myringitis typically presents with symptoms similar to acute otitis media. However, it can be differentiated from otitis media by physical examination, which is significant for vesicles on the eardrum (Fig. 1.13). Inflammation is typically limited to the tympanic membrane and the immediately adjacent external ear canal. Although mycoplasma pneumonia has been described as a

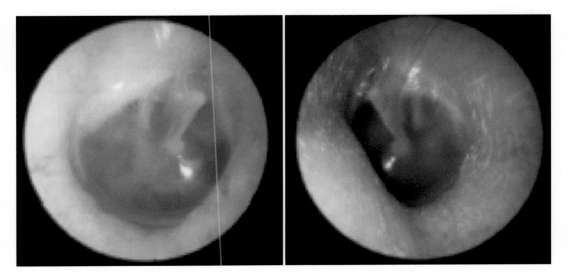

Fig. 1.9 Normal view of a right and left tympanic membrane (courtesy of Gerald Zahtz, MD)

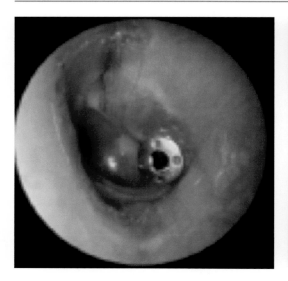

Fig. 1.10 Pressure-equalizing tube in place—left ear (courtesy of Gerald Zahtz, MD)

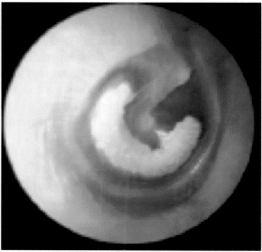

Fig. 1.12 Tympanic membrane with tympanosclerosis—right ear (courtesy of Gerald Zahtz, MD)

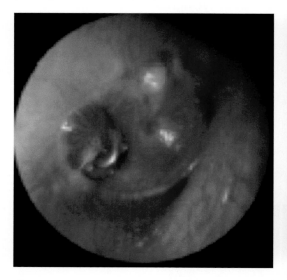

Fig. 1.11 Granulation tissue around pressure-equalizing tube—right ear (courtesy of Gerald Zahtz, MD)

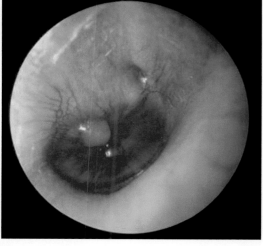

Fig. 1.13 Bullous myringitis—left ear (reprinted from the Hawke Library [hawkelibrary.com]; with permission)

rare etiologic agent, bullous myringitis is most commonly considered to be viral in origin [18]. Treatment is similar to acute otitis media.

Tympanic Membrane Perforation

Tympanic membrane perforations occur quite commonly in the pediatric population (Fig. 1.14).

Perforations occur for a variety of reasons and may be iatrogenic following tympanostomy tube placement [19, 20]. Other etiologies include acute or chronic otitis media and trauma such as blunt head trauma or blast injury [21]. Small perforations typically do not cause significant hearing loss or symptoms, but larger perforations can. Treatment involves patching the perforated eardrum, and surgical options range

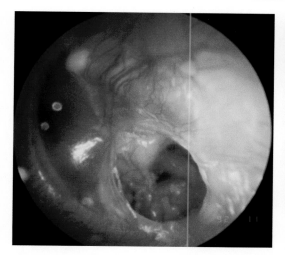

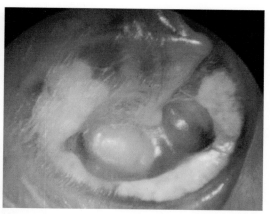

Fig. 1.15 Grade 3 atelectatic tympanic membrane—right ear (courtesy of Gerald Zahtz, MD)

Fig. 1.14 Tympanic membrane perforation—left ear (courtesy of Gerald Zahtz, MD)

from myringoplasty for small perforations to medial and lateral graft tympanoplasty techniques for larger perforations.

Atelectasis

Tympanic atelectasis is a frequently encountered problem in pediatrics and is related to Eustachian tube dysfunction and negative middle ear pressure. It refers to displacement of the tympanic membrane medially toward the promontory. It varies in severity and was classified based on severity by Sade in 1976 [22]. Grade 1 atelectasis refers to a mild retraction of the tympanic membrane only; if the tympanic membrane is retracted to the point of contact with the incus or stapes, it is defined as a grade 2 atelectasis. Grade 3 is defined as a tympanic membrane that makes contact with but is not adhered to the promontory (Fig. 1.15), and grade 4 refers to a tympanic membrane that is adhered to the promontory, also known as adhesive otitis media (Fig. 1.16).

Tympanic Cholesteatoma

As a result of a prior tympanoplasty or tympanostomy tube, squamous debris can be trapped and

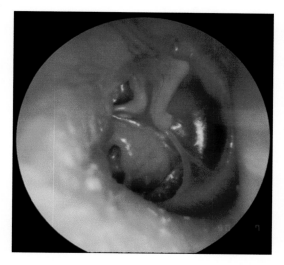

Fig. 1.16 Grade 4 atelectatic tympanic membrane; adhesive otitis media—right ear (courtesy of Gerald Zahtz, MD)

develop into an iatrogenic, intratympanic cholesteatoma (Fig. 1.17) that appears on examination as a keratin pearl along the tympanic membrane [23].

Middle Ear

The middle ear is the air-filled portion of the ear located medial to the eardrum and lateral to the oval window and round window of the internal ear. The ossicles are housed within the middle ear and are crucial for sound transduction from the

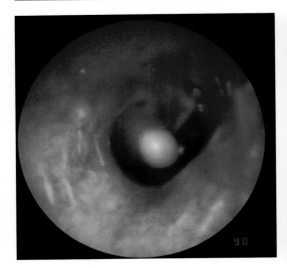

Fig. 1.17 Intratympanic cholesteatoma—right ear (courtesy of Gerald Zahtz, MD)

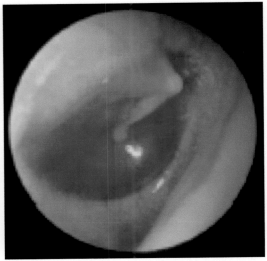

Fig. 1.18 Serous middle ear effusion—right ear (courtesy of Gerald Zahtz, MD)

external ear to the inner ear; therefore, pathology involving the middle ear space frequently results in decreased hearing. The Eustachian tube provides a connection from the middle ear space into the nasopharynx and is important for pressure equalization between the middle ear and throat; dysfunction of the Eustachian tube can result in a variety of middle ear diseases.

Middle Ear Effusion

Middle ear effusions can be acute or chronic and may consist of isolated or mixed serous, mucoid, and/or purulent fluid. Figure 1.18 demonstrates a serous middle ear effusion of a right ear. A serous effusion can also be accompanied by air bubbles (Fig. 1.19). Figure 1.20 demonstrates a purulent middle ear effusion, and Fig. 1.21 demonstrates a mucoid middle ear effusion. Acute effusions are often associated with middle ear infections, such as acute otitis media, whereas chronic effusions are typically attributed to Eustachian tube dysfunction.

Congenital Cholesteatoma

Congenital cholesteatoma is a diagnosis that pertains exclusively to the pediatric population—these cholesteatomas are defined as

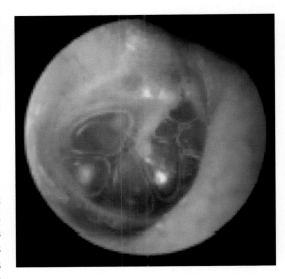

Fig. 1.19 Serous middle ear effusion with air bubbles—right ear (courtesy of Gerald Zahtz, MD)

occurring in patients with no prior history of otorrhea, tympanic perforation, or previous otologic procedure; on examination patients have a normal pars tensa and pars flaccida [24]. A white pearly mass that represents the cholesteatoma is visualized medial to the tympanic membrane. Figure 1.22 illustrates a congenital cholesteatoma of the right ear with a well-ventilated middle ear space.

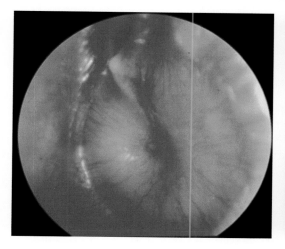

Fig. 1.20 Purulent middle ear effusion—left ear (courtesy of Gerald Zahtz, MD)

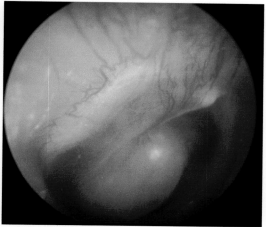

Fig. 1.22 Congenital cholesteatoma—right ear (courtesy of Gerald Zahtz, MD)

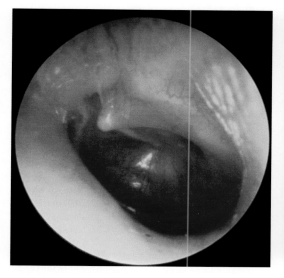

Fig. 1.21 Mucoid middle ear effusion—left ear (courtesy of Gerald Zahtz, MD)

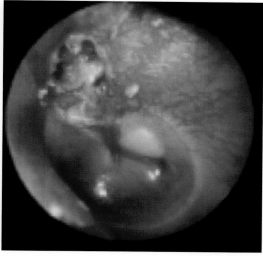

Fig. 1.23 Attic cholesteatoma—left ear (courtesy of Gerald Zahtz, MD)

Acquired Cholesteatoma

Acquired cholesteatoma occurs in ears with a history of middle ear disease or surgical intervention such as myringotomy with tubes or tympanoplasty. Unlike congenital cholesteatoma, the eardrum is typically not intact, and the disease tends to be much more difficult to manage [25].

A primary acquired cholesteatoma occurs as a retraction pocket, usually located in the pars flaccida, that enlarges and collects keratin debris; the underlying pathology is Eustachian tube dysfunction. Endoscopic examination typically reveals an intact pars tensa with a retraction pocket in the pars flaccida, the depths of which cannot be fully visualized (Fig. 1.23). When limited

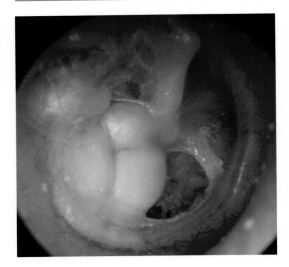

Fig. 1.24 Secondary acquired cholesteatoma with perforation—right ear (courtesy of Gerald Zahtz, MD)

to the attic, the disease is commonly referred to as attic cholesteatomas. Secondary acquired cholesteatoma originates from a tympanic membrane perforation; it is thought that as the edges of the tympanic membrane perforation try to heal, the squamous epithelium migrates into the middle ear. An example of a secondary acquired cholesteatoma with a visible perforation can be seen in Fig. 1.24. Although the underlying mechanisms differ, the disease process in primary and secondary acquired cholesteatoma progresses very similarly [26].

References

1. Karmody CS, Annino Jr DJ. Embryology and anomalies of the external ear. Facial Plast Surg. 1995;11:251–6.
2. Pecorari G, Tavormina P, Riva G, Landolfo V, Raimondo L, Garzaro M. Ear, nose and throat foreign bodies: the experience of the Pediatric Hospital of Turin. J Paediatr Child Health. 2014;50:978–84.
3. Balbani AP, Sanchez TG, Butugan O, Kii MA, Angélico Jr FV, Ikino CM, et al. Ear and nose foreign body removal in children. Int J Pediatr Otorhinolaryngol. 1998;46:37–42.
4. Schaefer P, Baugh RF. Acute otitis externa: an update. Am Fam Physician. 2012;86:1055–61.
5. McWilliams CJ, Smith CH, Goldman RD. Acute otitis externa in children. Can Fam Physician. 2012;58:1222–4.
6. Pontes ZB, Silva AD, Lima Ede O, Guerra Mde H, Oliveira NM, Carvalho Mde F, et al. Otomycosis: a retrospective study. Braz J Otorhinolaryngol. 2009;75:367–70.
7. Anwar K, Gohar MS. Otomycosis; clinical features, predisposing factors and treatment implications. Pak J Med Sci. 2014;30:564–7.
8. Carbone PN, Nelson BL. External auditory osteoma. Head Neck Pathol. 2012;6:244–6.
9. Hempel JM et al. Surgery for outer ear canal exostoses and osteomata: focusing on patient benefit and health-related quality of life. Otol Neurotol. 2012;33:83–6.
10. Wang C, Wu Y. The relationship between the ear protective measures and the prevalence of external auditory canal exostoses. Lin Chung Er Bi Yan Hou Tou Jing Wai Ke Za Zhi. 2014;28:1490–1.
11. Xenellis J, Mountricha A, Maragoudakis P, Kandiloros D, Assimakopoulos D, Linthicum FJ, et al. A histological examination in the cases of initial diagnosis as chronic otitis media with a polypoid mass in the external ear canal. Auris Nasus Larynx. 2011;38:325–8.
12. Eksan MS, Noorizan Y, Chew YK, Noorafidah MD, Asma A. Rare embryonal rhabdomyosarcoma of external acoustic canal: a case report and literature review. Am J Otolaryngol. 2014;35:814–5.
13. Farmer-Fedor BL, Rabbitt RD. Acoustic intensity, impedance and reflection coefficient in the human ear canal. J Acoust Soc Am. 2002;112:600–20.
14. Withnell RH, Gowdy LE. An analysis of the acoustic input impedance of the ear. J Assoc Res Otolaryngol. 2013;14:611–22.
15. Lim DJ. Structure and function of the tympanic membrane: a review. Acta Otorhinolaryngol Belg. 1995;49:101–15.
16. Gaihede M, Lildholdt T, Lunding J. Sequelae of secretory otitis media: changes in middle ear biomechanics. Acta Otolaryngol. 1997;117:382–9.
17. Siegel B, Chi DH. Contemporary guidelines for tympanostomy tube placement. Curr Treat Options Pediatr. 2015;1:234–41.
18. Cramer L, Emara DM, Gadre AK. Mycoplasma an unlikely cause of bullous myringitis. Ear Nose Throat J. 2012;91:E30–1.
19. O'Niel MB, Cassidy LD, Link TR, Kerschner JE. Tracking tympanostomy tube outcomes in pediatric patients with otitis media using an electronic database. Int J Pediatr Otorhinolaryngol. 2015;79:1275–8.
20. Adkins AP, Friedman EM. Surgical indications and outcomes of tympanostomy tube removal. Int J Pediatr Otorhinolaryngol. 2005;69:1047–51.
21. Quintana DA, Parker JR, Jordan FB, Tuggle DW, Mantor PC, Tunell WP. The spectrum of pediatric injuries after a bomb blast. J Pediatr Surg. 1997;32:307–10. discussion 310–1.
22. Sade J, Berco E. Atelectasis and secretory otitis media. Ann Otol Rhinol Laryngol. 1976;85(2 Suppl 25 Pt 2):66–72.

23. Atmaca S, Seckin E, Koyuncu M. Tympanic membrane cholesteatoma: a rare finding. Turk J Pediatr. 2010;52:309–11.

24. Kazahaya K, Potsic WP. Congenital cholesteatoma. Curr Opin Otolaryngol Head Neck Surg. 2004;12: 398–403.

25. Morita Y, Yamamoto Y, Oshima S, Takahashi K, Takahashi S. Pediatric middle ear cholesteatoma: the comparative study of congenital cholesteatoma and acquired cholesteatoma. Eur Arch Otorhinolaryngol. 2015 June 5. [Epub ahead of print].

26. Vikram BK, Udayashankar SG, Naseeruddin K, Venkatesha BK, Manjunath D, Savantrewwa IR. Complications in primary and secondary acquired cholesteatoma: a prospective comparative study of 62 ears. Am J Otolaryngol. 2008;29:1–6.

Nasal Cavity and Nasopharynx

2

Nathan Gonik and Elena B. Willis Woodson

Nasal Cavity

The nasal cavities are individual chambers separated by the midline septum (Fig. 2.1) and joined posteriorly in the nasopharynx. The septum is cartilaginous anteriorly and caudally and joins the ethmoid, palate, and maxilla posteriorly. It is lined with respiratory mucosa. Three outpouchings of bone and highly vascularized mucosa divide the nasal airway further. The superior turbinate rests above the superior meatus, the middle turbinate rests above the middle meatus, and the inferior turbinate covers the inferior meatus.

The nasolacrimal duct runs from the lacrimal fossa to the inferior meatus. Sitting behind the uncinate process, the frontal, maxillary, and ethmoid sinuses open into the middle meatus. Behind the superior turbinate, the posterior ethmoid and sphenoid cells drain into the spheno-ethmoidal recess. The nasal cavity is bounded by the skull base superiorly and the orbits superiorly and laterally.

N. Gonik, M.D., M.H.S.A. (✉)
Department of Otolaryngology, Wayne State
University School of Medicine, Children's Hospital
of Michigan, Detroit, MI, USA
e-mail: ngonik@dmc.org

E.B.W. Woodson, M.D.
Otolaryngology and Audiology, Oklahoma
University, Oklahoma City, OK, USA
e-mail: elenabethwillis@gmail.com

Acute Rhinosinusitis

Acute rhinosinusitis is a clinical diagnosis that is often hard to distinguish from an uncomplicated upper respiratory tract infection (URI) [4]. Simple URIs have more mild symptoms that are often associated with a systemic viral syndrome. In general, the most severe symptoms of a viral URI (including fever and myalgias) should begin abating after 24–48 h, even if purulent nasal secretions are present. The presumptive diagnosis of acute bacterial rhinosinusitis is made when any of the following criteria are met:

1. Persistent illness with nasal discharge and/or daytime cough lasting longer than 10 days
2. Worsening course of nasal discharge, daytime cough, or fever after initial improvement
3. Severe onset of concurrent purulent nasal discharge and fever at least 39 °C for at least 3 consecutive days

For persistent illness, observation is recommended until at least 10 days after the onset of symptoms, because many of these illnesses will resolve spontaneously. For worsening or severe presentations, treatment with antibiotics is recommended and generally involves amoxicillin with or without clavulanic acid. Cultures are generally not necessary but can be considered for persistent disease after appropriate therapy to help direct further treatment (Fig. 2.2).

© Springer International Publishing Switzerland 2016
J. Cheng, J.P. Bent (eds.), *Endoscopic Atlas of Pediatric Otolaryngology*,
DOI 10.1007/978-3-319-29471-1_2

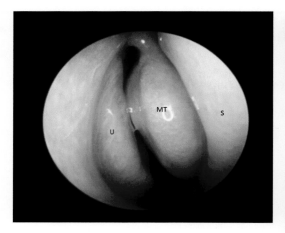

Fig. 2.1 Normal nasal endoscopy. *MT* middle turbinate, *S* septum, *U* uncinate process

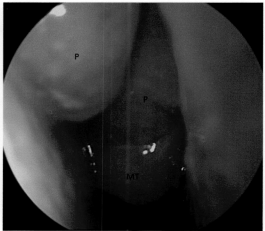

Fig. 2.3 Chronic rhinosinusitis with polyposis. Mucosal edema and polypoid degeneration of mucosa obscure and obstruct normal anatomy. *MT* middle turbinate, *P* polyp

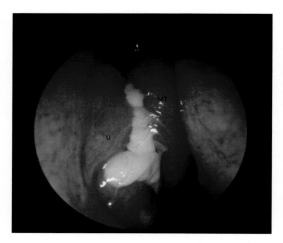

Fig. 2.2 Acute bacterial rhinosinusitis. Inflamed middle turbinate (MT) and uncinate process (U) with purulence draining from the middle meatus (reprinted from the Hawke Library [hawkelibrary.com]; with permission)

Chronic Rhinosinusitis

Chronic rhinosinusitis (CRS) refers to inflammation of the sinonasal tract for at least 12 weeks. The four cardinal symptoms of CRS are mucopurulent drainage, nasal obstruction, facial pain/pressure, and hyposmia [5]. Generally, at least two of these symptoms must be present and accompanied by computed tomography (CT) or endoscopic evidence of mucosal inflammation for a definitive diagnosis (Fig. 2.3). CRS can be further subdivided into CRS with polyposis, CRS

without polyposis, and allergic fungal sinusitis (AFS). AFS is characterized by the presence of allergic mucin—thick inspissated secretions with eosinophils and fungal hyphae [6].

In any child with sinonasal polyposis or recalcitrant CRS, cystic fibrosis (CF), ciliary dyskinesia, and immunodeficiency should be considered. CF is caused by an autosomal recessive mutation in the cystic fibrosis transmembrane regulator (CFTR) gene that controls the passage of chloride and bicarbonate ions [7]. Thickened secretions and bacterial colonization impair mucociliary clearance and lead to CRS in nearly all CF patients and polyps in more than 80 % of individuals (Fig. 2.4).

Treatment for chronic sinusitis is divided into medical and surgical options. Generally, surgery is considered only after maximal medical management has failed. Nasal saline irrigations may help clear inflammatory debris and dried secretions that obstruct the natural flow of mucous. Topical nasal steroids and oral antihistamines decrease the local inflammatory response and decrease mucosal edema. While it is important to limit antibiotic use for acute viral infections, there is considerable evidence supporting their use in CRS. Prolonged courses of antibiotics covering both gram-positive and gram-negative organisms should be considered before proceeding to surgery [8].

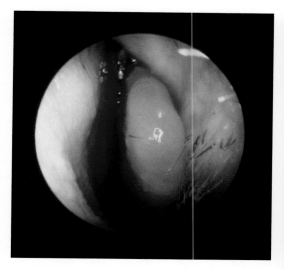

Fig. 2.4 Polyposis with cystic fibrosis. Extensive polyps extending into the nasal vestibule obstructing nasal drainage and airflow (reprinted from the Hawke Library [hawkelibrary.com]; with permission)

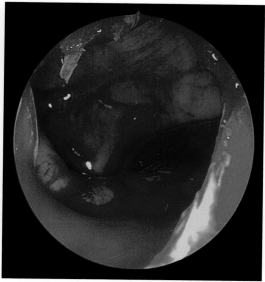

Fig. 2.5 Maxillary antrostomy. Endoscopic view of the maxillary sinus through a large antrostomy

An area where pediatric and adult CRS differ is in the management of the adenoids. The adenoid bed can harbor bacterial biofilms that are difficult to eradicate with antibiotics and act as a nidus for chronic infections [9]. Adenoidectomy is one of the most frequent pediatric surgeries and is much quicker than sinus surgery. Many otolaryngologists will consider adenoidectomy prior to pediatric endoscopic sinus surgery [10]. When discussing endoscopic sinus surgery, some surgeons advocate for large antrostomies to allow maximum ventilation of sinuses (Fig. 2.5). Others advocate for balloon dilation, partial uncinectomy, or smaller antrostomies to minimize interference with bony growth of the midface [11, 12].

Allergic Fungal Rhinosinusitis

Allergic fungal rhinosinusitis (AFRS) is diagnosed by the presence of mucosal inflammation with allergic mucin containing fungal hyphal elements. Allergic mucin is characterized by thick, tenacious mucous containing fungal elements, necrotic inflammatory cells, eosinophils, and Charcot-Leyden crystals. Some require elevated serum IgE to fungi as a critical diagnostic factor.

If elevated, it tends to suggest poor local immunity in the sinonasal tract and a more difficult therapeutic course [13]. AFRS is often considered a sinus manifestation of allergic bronchopulmonary aspergillosis. Consequently, patients often present with multiple atopic complaints, including allergic reactions and asthma or other reactive airway diseases.

Endoscopically, anatomy may be altered by dense polypoid changes to the mucosa. Due to the chronic accumulation of allergic mucin, the sinus cavities may be expanded with thinned or eroded surrounding bone (Figs. 2.6, 2.7, and 2.8). Even after the sinus cavities have been exposed and opened surgically, the tenacious mucin can stick to surrounding tissue, making removal difficult. Irrigation with or without pressured instruments may be necessary to clear the debris.

Treatment must include nasal lavage and topical steroids to improve sinus outflow and remove inflammatory debris. Systemic steroids may be beneficial, particularly during exacerbations and preoperatively. Systemic and topical antifungals have a more controversial role, and there is no adequate evidence at this time to strongly support or reject their use [14, 15].

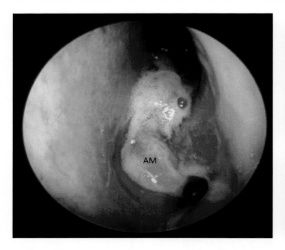

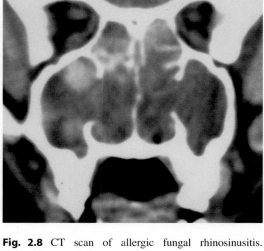

Fig. 2.6 Allergic fungal rhinosinusitis. Polypoid mucosal changes with thick allergic mucin filling the nasal cavity (reprinted from the Hawke Library [hawkelibrary.com]; with permission)

Fig. 2.8 CT scan of allergic fungal rhinosinusitis. Polypoid mucosal changes and expanded maxillary sinuses filled with dense heterogeneous contents (reprinted from the Hawke Library [hawkelibrary.com]; with permission)

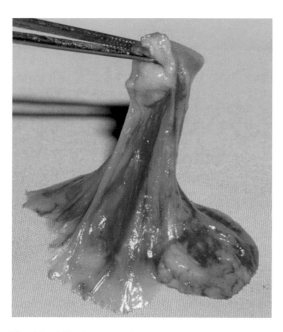

Fig. 2.7 Allergic mucin. Tenacious allergic mucin is difficult to manipulate due to its concentrated, sticky nature (reprinted from the Hawke Library [hawkelibrary.com]; with permission)

nates are covered in respiratory mucosa and, similar to the sinus cavities, can be impacted by acute or chronic inflammatory reactions affecting the entire airway. Histologically, turbinate hypertrophy is caused by enlargement of the medial mucosal layer and lamina propria as they undergo fibrosis and proliferate with venous sinuses and inflammatory cells [16]. This explains the characteristic pale or boggy appearance seen in patients with allergic and nonallergic rhinosinusitis (Figs. 2.9 and 2.10). All turbinates can become hypertrophied; however, the inferior turbinate is most visible at the nasal orifice and is commonly implicated in nasal airway obstruction (Fig. 2.11). Treatment is similar to that for CRS and typically begins with nasal hygiene and topical steroids. There are many surgical techniques to remove portions of the turbinate to increase airflow. These can be divided into turbinate reduction procedures, where the submucosal tissue is removed by ablation or excision, and partial turbinectomy, where portions of the bone and mucosa are removed.

Turbinate Hypertrophy

Turbinate hypertrophy can present as a solitary finding or together with other pathologies like chronic sinusitis or septal deviation. The turbi-

Concha Bullosa

Because the middle turbinate is a bony projection of the ethmoid bone, it too can become aerated similar to other ethmoidal air cells (Figs. 2.12

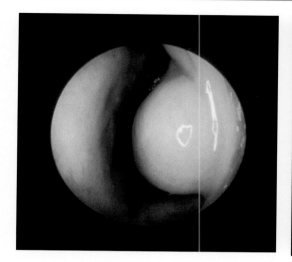

Fig. 2.9 Inferior turbinate hypertrophy. Hypertrophic inferior turbinate with characteristic pale mucosa

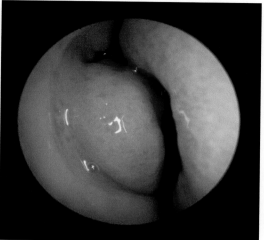

Fig. 2.11 Fibrotic inferior turbinate. Fibrotic mucosal changes in a large and obstructive inferior turbinate suggesting chronic hypertrophic and inflammatory changes (reprinted from the Hawke Library [hawkelibrary.com]; with permission)

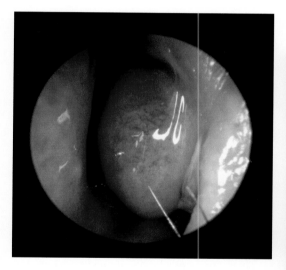

Fig. 2.10 Boggy inferior turbinate. Inferior turbinate with thick secretions suggestive of chronic inflammation and venous dilation

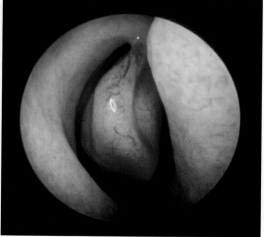

Fig. 2.12 Concha bullosa. Partially pneumatized middle turbinate demonstrating normal anatomy anteriorly and aeration posteriorly (reprinted from the Hawke Library [hawkelibrary.com]; with permission)

and 2.13). This occurs in approximately 45 % of individuals and is often an incidental finding [17]. The middle turbinate rests over the hiatus semilunaris and the ostia of the frontal, maxillary, and anterior ethmoid sinuses. As the turbinate enlarges and aerates, it can occlude sinus outflow or fill with secretions [18]. If secretions become trapped in the concha, a mucocele or mucopyocele can develop. This can be a source of pain, persistent infection, and chronic sinus disease. If

symptomatic, surgical approaches involve marsupializing the air cell into the nasal cavity while preserving the structure of the middle turbinate. Other bony landmarks can also become pneumatized, including the uncinate bone and superior turbinate. The middle turbinate concha bullosa is more common.

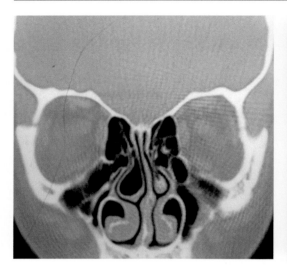

Fig. 2.13 Concha bullosa. CT scan demonstrating pneumatized right middle turbinate obstructing and filling the middle meatus (reprinted from the Hawke Library [hawkelibrary.com]; with permission)

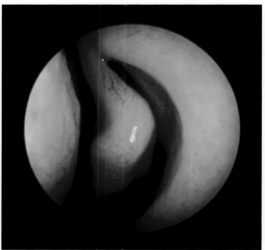

Fig. 2.14 Paradoxical middle turbinate. S-shaped middle turbinate with lateral convexity (reprinted from the Hawke Library [hawkelibrary.com]; with permission)

Paradoxical Middle Turbinate

The term "paradoxical" middle turbinate (PMT) refers to an aberrant curvature of the middle turbinate bone. As opposed to a normal C-shaped turbinate with a lateral concavity, the PMT is typically S-shaped with a large lateral convexity (Fig. 2.14). The pathological significance of this finding is often debated. Approximately 25 % of individuals will have PMT as an incidental finding; however, the presence of a PMT does not seem to predispose to acute or CRS [19]. If the turbinate is thought to be obstructive on endoscopy, partial excision to improve the patency and outflow of the middle meatus is recommended [20].

Septal Deviation

While the symptoms and complaints are generally simple, the anatomic source of nasal obstruction in a child can be difficult to determine. Nasal septal deviation (NSD) is often missed, as attention may be directed at the turbinates or nasopharynx during endoscopy. Additionally, turbinate and adenoid hypertrophy can, and often do, coexist with NSD. This highlights the need

for detailed anterior rhinoscopy prior to attempts at instrumentation or decongestion. Dynamic collapse of the nasal valves can help guide the exam, and often the best view is attained without a telescope or speculum (Fig. 2.15).

The prevalence of NSD is a matter of debate and, depending on the age in question, can range from 2 to 90 % [21]. Some attribute pediatric NSD to nasal trauma in utero, during delivery, or throughout life. Others suggest that it is caused by genetic predisposition or differential growth patterns in the facial skeleton. Along with nasal obstruction, some authors attribute chronic sinus and middle ear disease to NSD [22].

There are many classification systems used to describe septal deviation quantitatively and qualitatively. It is often best to utilize by describing the shape (S-shaped, C-shaped, spur), location (anterior/posterior, superior/inferior), laterality, and severity (Figs. 2.16 and 2.17). Passing an endoscope beyond an initial deviated segment may identify additional pathology and should be attempted when possible. While surgery can be attempted on patients of any age, most surgeons will defer septal surgery until the patient reaches 12–14 years of age due to concerns for altering bony-cartilaginous growth centers. This topic is very controversial, and the choice of when to

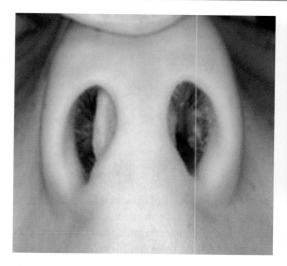

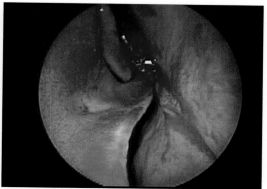

Fig. 2.17 Septal spur. Septal deviation caused by a bony spur of the maxillary crest extending into the middle meatus

Fig. 2.15 Caudal nasal septal deviation. Anterior rhinoscopy visualizing a caudal septal deviation to the right. Endoscopy or speculum exams could miss this finding because they do not permit a view until positioned in the nasal vestibule

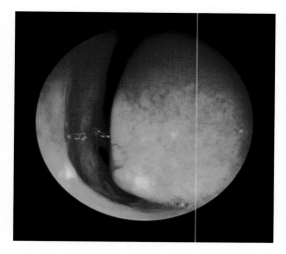

Fig. 2.16 Nasal septal deviation. Endoscopic view of a right-sided, severe, C-shaped deformity of the septum (reprinted from the Hawke Library [hawkelibrary.com]; with permission)

operate will depend on the severity of an individual patient's complaints and presentation.

Foreign Body

Nasal foreign bodies are commonly encountered in otolaryngology and emergency room visits. Presentations may be explicit, with a clear history of nasal insertion, or more subtle, with reports of facial pain, nasal obstruction, foul smell, and/or nasal drainage. Any object that can fit into the nasal orifice can be inserted. The most common foreign bodies are beads, followed by toys and paper objects [23]. Aside from nasal obstruction, foreign bodies may pose additional risks necessitating early removal. The nasal cavity communicates directly with the pharynx, and it is possible to aspirate foreign bodies if they migrate posteriorly. Additionally, some foreign bodies, particularly watch or button batteries, cause erosions or burns to the surrounding soft tissue. This can lead to mucosal injury, scarring, or destruction of the bony-cartilaginous nasal cavity. A critical component of the nasal foreign body endoscopic examination involves examining the contralateral cavity and reexamining the nasal cavity after foreign body removal, always being prepared for a second foreign body, especially in younger children and poor historians (Fig. 2.18).

Antrochoanal Polyp

Antrochoanal polyps originate in the maxillary sinus and extend through the sinus ostia, under the middle turbinate (Fig. 2.19). They can grow quite large and extend into or beyond the nasopharynx. Although often coexisting with CRS, they differ from diffuse nasal polyposis in that they are typically unilateral and encountered at a younger age [24]. Depending on the size and

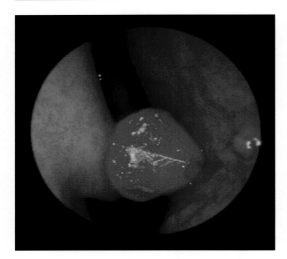

Fig. 2.18 Nasal foreign body. A bead is encountered between the septum and the inferior turbinate (reprinted from the Hawke Library [hawkelibrary.com]; with permission)

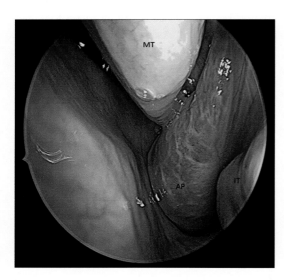

Fig. 2.19 Antrochoanal polyp. Polyp extending from the ostium of the maxillary sinus, under the middle turbinate, and into the nasopharynx

extent of the polyp, patients may present with nasal obstruction or a variety of pharyngeal concerns, including voice changes, cough, or globus sensation. There is no known etiology; however, microscopically they resemble retention cysts with exuberant inflammatory polyp formation [25]. Surgical approaches can be

either endonasal or open. Simple polyp excision will often lead to recurrence if the point of origin within the sinus is not addressed. Depending on the polyp's insertion, a Caldwell-Luc approach may be necessary to achieve complete excision.

Epistaxis

Epistaxis is a common pediatric complaint. The most common cause of epistaxis is nasal trauma. Sports, falls, vehicular accidents, and digital manipulation can cause mucosal disruption that leads to bleeding from the highly vascular nasal mucosa. Bleeding can also be caused by excessive dryness often seen during winter months, when there is less ambient humidity due to freezing temperatures and home heating. Most epistaxis is self-limited and is caused by bleeding from Kiesselbach's plexus in Little's area (Fig. 2.20). The plexus is fed by four named arteries and its location, in the partially exposed nasal vestibule, predisposing the area to high risk of drying and trauma. Direct pressure, applied by collapsing the nasal ala for 5–15 min, should resolve most anterior bleeds.

Posterior epistaxis describes an arterial bleed from a branch of the sphenopalatine artery. This can be more difficult to control because it is not accessible via external pressure. When external pressure fails to resolve epistaxis, topical hemostatic agents or nasal packing is required. The pediatric endoscopic exam during an acute bleed is rarely helpful except in the operative setting; the nasal cavity will fill with blood unless there is adequate suction. Endoscopy is more useful in the patient with chronic or recurrent epistaxis and may be necessary to identify excoriated mucosa, dilated nasal vessels, septal perforations, angiofibromas, or other anomalies. If bleeding is generally easily controlled and not life threatening, humidification with saline gels or other emollients can be beneficial. Cauterizing potential bleeding sources may be necessary as well. For recalcitrant or life-threatening bleeding, laboratory and radiologic tests may be necessary to rule out and treat coagulopathies and vascular lesions.

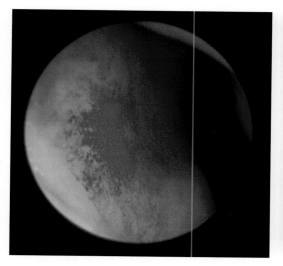

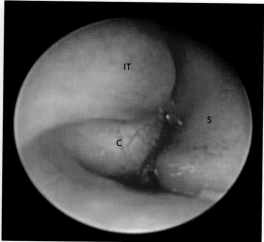

Fig. 2.20 Epistaxis. Hyperemia and injection of the anterior septum representing bleeding from Kiesselbach's plexus

Fig. 2.21 Nasolacrimal duct cyst. Cyst (C) emerging from underneath the inferior turbinate (IT) obstructing the nasal cavity in a neonate. *S* septum

Nasolacrimal Duct Cyst

Nasolacrimal duct cysts are an uncommon cause of infantile nasal obstruction. Approximately 30 % of infants are born with nasolacrimal duct obstruction that will eventually resolve [26]. A small fraction of these patients will develop a cyst at the inferior end of the nasolacrimal duct. Endoscopically this can be seen as a cystic outpouching emerging from underneath the inferior turbinate (Fig. 2.21). When a nasolacrimal duct cyst causes obstruction of the nasal cavity and respiratory distress, it can be marsupialized surgically via an endoscopic approach. Occasionally, dacryocystorhinostomy may also be required to cannulate a tract between the lacrimal sac and the nasal cavity.

Piriform Aperture Stenosis

Piriform aperture stenosis (PAS) is a narrowing of the nasal inlet caused by a local dysostosis of the maxilla. PAS can manifest as a solitary anomaly or in conjunction with other congenital defects in the same developmental field. It is often seen in conjunction with holoprosencephaly and a congenital midline mega-incisor.

Children present with varying degrees of nasal obstruction in the early neonatal period. Cyclical patterns of respiratory distress with difficulty feeding and relief while crying are typical. Attempts to pass an endoscope will often fail when a shelf at the piriform aperture is encountered (Figs. 2.22 and 2.23). Because these infants are obligate nasal breathers, PAS represents a potential medical emergency. Initial attempts to stabilize respiration include nasal decongestants, irrigation, and steroids, while supplemental oxygen can be delivered via a nasal cannula or an oral airway. If the child cannot be successfully weaned from supplemental oxygen, surgical correction via a sublabial incision with postoperative stenting may be required [27]. The differential diagnosis includes neonatal rhinitis, nasolacrimal duct cyst, and choanal atresia. A maxillofacial CT scan demonstrating a piriform aperture smaller than 11 mm is diagnostic.

Granulomatosis with Polyangiitis (Wegener's Granulomatosis)

Granulomatosis with polyangiitis (GPA), previously referred to as Wegener's granulomatosis, is a systemic vasculitis characterized by the presence

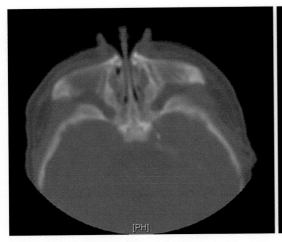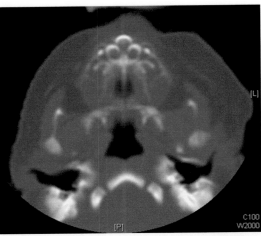

Fig. 2.22 Piriform aperture stenosis (PAS). Axial CT scans demonstrating local dysostosis at the piriform aperture, narrowing the nasal cavity (**a**), and a central mega maxillary incisor (**b**), a common feature associated with PAS (courtesy of Lee Smith, MD, New Hyde Park, NY)

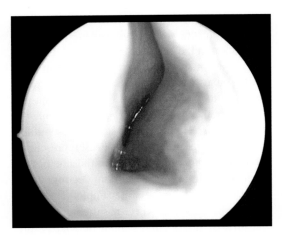

Fig. 2.23 Piriform aperture stenosis. Inability to pass the endoscope beyond the narrowing in a patient with piriform aperture stenosis (courtesy of Lee Smith, MD, New Hyde Park, NY)

Endoscopically, extensive crusting with areas of erosion and scarring are typically encountered (Fig. 2.24). Diagnosis can be made serologically or via biopsy of involved mucosa. Endoscopic sinus surgery can be difficult in GPA patients due to altered anatomy and scarring of normal anatomic structures. In addition to surgery for chronic sinusitis and epistaxis, the inferior meatus may become obstructed, necessitating surgical correction of uncontrolled epiphora. Conservative measures include nasal lavage and humidification to minimize crust formation and prolonged courses of topical steroids and antibiotics as needed. Management with immune suppression can improve systemic and sinonasal manifestations of the disease [30]. Close follow-up and medical management from rheumatology services is recommended.

Choanal Atresia

Choanal atresia occurs when there is no communication between the nasal cavity and the nasopharynx. It is relatively rare, occurring in 1:5000 to 1:8000 live births annually. When it is unilateral, it is often a solitary finding and may not be noticed until the child enters grade school and complains of nasal obstruction or chronic unilateral discharge. Bilateral choanal atresia is an

of necrotizing granulomas and C-ANCA serum positivity. Most patients (72–99 %) with GPA will have head and neck involvement at some point in their lives [28]. Sinonasal manifestations are present in approximately 85 % of patients. Of those, chronic crusting and rhinosinusitis are the most common complaints, followed by nasal obstruction and bloody discharge [29]. The disease can progress to septal erosion and cosmetic deformities.

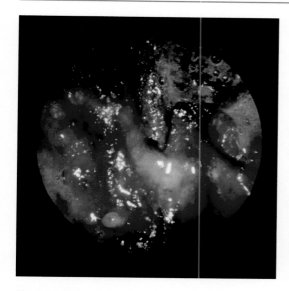

Fig. 2.24 Wegener's granulomatosis of the nasal cavity. Extensive crusting along the septum

emergency in the neonatal period because the infant is an obligate nasal breather. Endoscopy may be difficult as secretions pool in the posterior nasal cavity (Fig. 2.25). Bilateral choanal atresia is often associated with other syndromes, including CHARGE, Pfeiffer, Apert, and Crouzon [31]. Surgical correction can be attempted endoscopically or via a transpalatal approach.

Nasopharynx

The pediatric nasopharynx is anatomically part of the pharynx, but functionally it serves as part of the respiratory system. The nasal portion of the pharynx undergoes changes during development. At birth it is quite narrow and gradually curves down to the oropharynx. By puberty the nasopharynx has widened and a right angle is seen at the nasopharyngeal-oropharyngeal junction. The adenoids are located on the roof and the Eustachian tubes lie on the lateral aspect of the nasopharynx. Examination of the nasopharynx is most often accomplished by flexible fiber-optic laryngoscopy. Radiographic examination with CT or magnetic resonance imaging (MRI) often provides important information about this relatively inaccessible region (Fig. 2.26) [32].

Adenoid Hypertrophy

In infants and children, the relatively small size of the nasopharynx and the large size of the peritubal lymphatic tissue (adenoids) can cause nasal and Eustachian tube obstruction [32]. Adenoid hypertrophy along with tonsillar hypertrophy is the most common cause of sleep-disordered breathing in children. Evaluation of adenoid size can be difficult in children. Fiber-optic endoscopy is often used to grade the size of adenoid tissue preoperatively. Parikh et al. developed a grading system that stages adenoid size (grades 1–4) based on anatomic structures that come in contact with the hypertrophied adenoid tissue (Figs. 2.27, 2.28, 2.29) [33–39]. Another method of evaluation is lateral neck radiographs; however, direct visualization by endoscopy has demonstrated better correlation with symptoms [40]. Removal of adenoid tissue can improve Eustachian tube dysfunction, nasal congestion, and sleep-disordered breathing in select patients. Removal can be performed in a variety of ways, including suction cautery, curette, and powered microdebrider.

Adenoiditis

Inflammation of the adenoid tissue, or adenoiditis, may be characterized by duration of symptoms as acute or chronic. Most cases of acute adenoiditis are associated with a viral illness during the winter months. Adenovirus, influenza virus, parainfluenza, and enteroviruses are the most common culprits. The infection is almost always self-limited and of short duration, showing improvement within 10 days [32]. In chronic adenoiditis, children are often colonized with *Haemophilus influenzae*, *Streptococcus pneumoniae*, *Streptococcus pyogenes*, and *Staphylococcus aureus* [33–39]. Sinonasal infection can occur more commonly in patients with enlarged adenoids due to stasis of secretions secondary to the obstruction [39]. Treatment of recurrent bacterial adenoiditis consists of oral antibiotics and possibly adenoidectomy in patients with persistent sinonasal complaints (Fig. 2.30) [32].

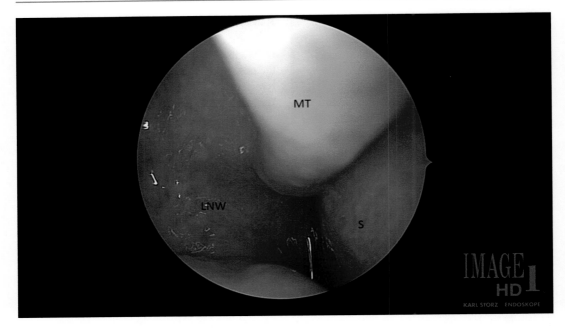

Fig. 2.25 Choanal atresia. Nasopharyngeal inlet obstructed by an atretic plate of bone and mucosa. Secretions pool at the junction of the lateral nasal wall (LNW) and the hypertrophic septum (S). *MT* middle turbinate

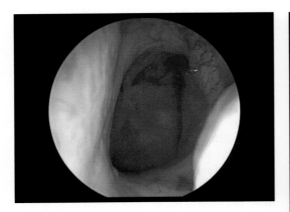

Fig. 2.26 Normal nasopharynx, 1+ adenoid hypertrophy

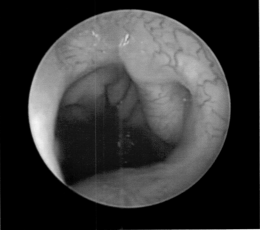

Fig. 2.27 Mild, 2+ adenoid hypertrophy

Velopharyngeal Insufficiency

The velopharyngeal sphincter comprises six muscles: the superior constrictor, palatopharyngeus, palatoglossus, levator veli palatini, tensor veli palatini, and musculus uvulae. Closure of the palate during speech is accomplished through the combined function of these muscles. Proper closure of the velopharynx is required to produce nonnasal consonant phonemes and vowels [32].

Causes of velopharyngeal insufficiency (VPI) include errors in speech production as well as structural and neuromuscular abnormalities. Cleft palate, submucous cleft, and adenoid removal are the most frequent causes of VPI [41, 42]. The most common syndrome associated with VPI is velocardiofacial syndrome. Evaluation of VPI includes speech and language assessment by an experienced speech-language pathologist as well as nasopharyngoscopy to evaluate palatal movement during speech. Treatment for VPI depends on severity of symptoms and often includes speech therapy, prosthetic devices, or surgical intervention with pharyngeal flaps, sphincter pharyngoplasty, palatoplasty, or posterior pharyngeal wall augmentation (Figs. 2.31 and 2.32).

Juvenile Nasopharyngeal Angiofibroma

Juvenile nasopharyngeal angiofibroma is a histologically benign tumor that can exhibit malignant and aggressive behavior and typically occurs in adolescent males. It arises at the sphenopalatine foramen and can be seen on nasal endoscopy at the posterior nasal cavity and nasopharynx. Depending on the extent of the tumor, endoscopic resection with ligation of the sphenopalatine artery is often the treatment of choice. Open operative approaches are also indicated in certain patients [43]. Staging of these tumors is important for surgical decision making and predicting recurrence and prognosis [44]. This is a highly vascular tumor that usually requires preoperative embolization for adequate hemostasis during resection (Figs. 2.33 and 2.34).

Rhabdomyosarcoma

Rhabdomyosarcoma is the most common soft-tissue tumor in children. Nasopharyngeal rhabdomyosarcomas tend to grow rapidly and invade adjacent structures (Fig. 2.35) [45].

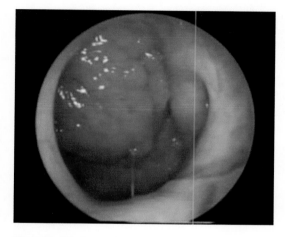

Fig. 2.28 Moderate, 3+ adenoid hypertrophy

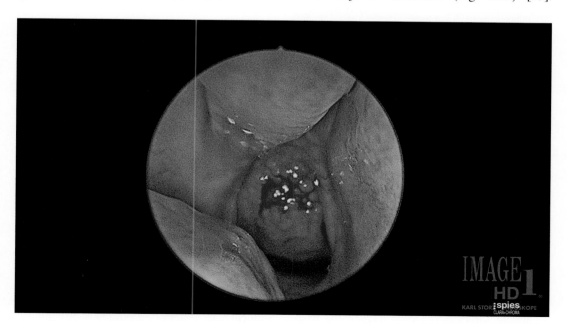

Fig. 2.29 Severe, 4+ adenoid hypertrophy

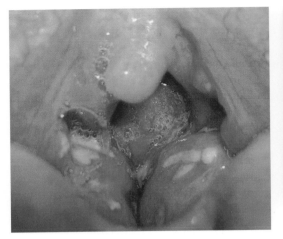

Fig. 2.30 Adenoiditis

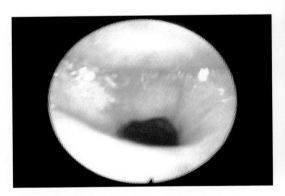

Fig. 2.31 Velopharyngeal insufficiency, circular closure

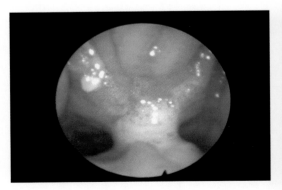

Fig. 2.32 Velopharyngeal insufficiency, narrow pharyngeal flap with persistent lateral gaps

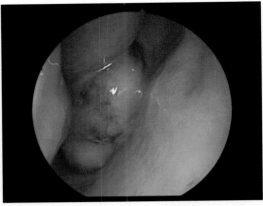

Fig. 2.33 Juvenile nasopharyngeal angiofibroma

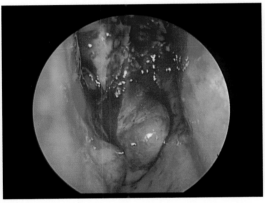

Fig. 2.34 Juvenile nasopharyngeal angiofibroma, intraoperative resection

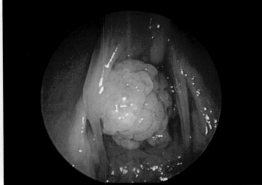

Fig. 2.35 Nasopharyngeal rhabdomyosarcoma

Treatment for rhabdomyosarcoma of the nasopharynx is multimodal therapy involving surgical resection, chemotherapy, and radiotherapy.

Surgical resection is often extremely difficult due to the inaccessibility of this area [46]. Chemotherapy in association with radiotherapy

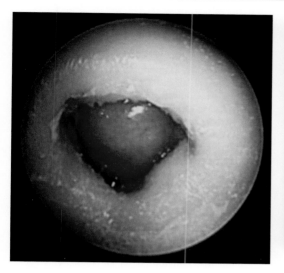

Fig. 2.36 Nasopharyngeal glioma

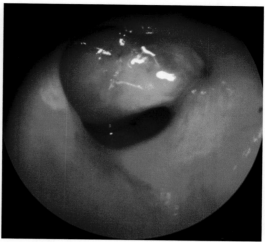

Fig. 2.37 Nasopharyngeal teratoma

has proven capable to obtain local and distant control of disease. Despite treatment, however, prognosis of relapsing disease remains poor [47].

Glioma

Nasopharyngeal glioma is a rare congenital malformation of neural origin (Fig. 2.36). It is thought to represent encephaloceles that become sequestered on the extracranial side of the skull base [48]. They often approximate skull base defects but lack communication to the subarachnoid space. Histologically, they contain mature neuroglial tissue and specialized central nervous system elements [49]. Neonates often present with nasal obstruction, which can be severe and life threatening. Radiographic imaging with MRI is indicated to assess for intracranial communication. Treatment is with surgical resection, including neurosurgical evaluation and intervention when appropriate.

Teratoma

Nasopharyngeal teratomas are rare neoplasms that are often present with respiratory distress in the neonate (Fig. 2.37) [50]. For safe management of these cases, prenatal evaluation, careful preoperative assessment of the airway, sufficient preparation, and intubation by an expert are essential [51]. The tumor comprises cystic and solid/fatty components and, often, calcifications. MRI can assist in the diagnosis of teratoma [32]. After stabilizing and securing the airway in these patients, complete surgical excision is the treatment of choice. Alpha-fetoprotein is an important tumor marker for detecting recurrence and residual disease [52].

References

1. Sasaki CT, Levine PA, Laitman JT, Crelin Jr ES. Postnatal descent of the epiglottis in man. A preliminary report. Arch Otolaryngol. 1977;103:169–71.
2. Park IH, Song JS, Choi H, Kim TH, Hoon S, Lee SH, et al. Volumetric study in the development of paranasal sinuses by CT imaging in Asian: a pilot study. Int J Pediatr Otorhinolaryngol. 2010;74:1347–50.
3. Isaac A, Major M, Witmans M, Alrajhi Y, Flores-Mir C, Major P, et al. Correlations between acoustic rhinometry, subjective symptoms, and endoscopic findings in symptomatic children with nasal obstruction. JAMA Otolaryngol Head Neck Surg. 2015;141:550–5.
4. Wald ER, Applegate KE, Bordley C, Darrow DH, Glode MP, Marcy SM, et al. Clinical practice guideline for the diagnosis and management of acute bacterial sinusitis in children aged 1 to 18 years. Pediatrics. 2013;132:e262–80.
5. Chan Y, Kuhn FA. An update on the classifications, diagnosis, and treatment of rhinosinusitis. Curr Opin Otolaryngol Head Neck Surg. 2009;17:204–8.

6. Bent 3rd JP, Kuhn FA. Diagnosis of allergic fungal sinusitis. Otolaryngol Head Neck Surg. 1994;111: 580–8.

7. Tandon R, Derkay C. Contemporary management of rhinosinusitis and cystic fibrosis. Curr Opin Otolaryngol Head Neck Surg. 2003;11:41–4.

8. Lusk R. Pediatric chronic rhinosinusitis. Curr Opin Otolaryngol Head Neck Surg. 2006;14:393–6.

9. Zuliani G, Carron M, Gurrola J, Coleman C, Haupert M, Berk R, et al. Identification of adenoid biofilms in chronic rhinosinusitis. Int J Pediatr Otorhinolaryngol. 2006;70:1613–7.

10. Sobol SE, Samadi DS, Kazahaya K, Tom LW. Trends in the management of pediatric chronic sinusitis: survey of the American Society of Pediatric Otolaryngology. Laryngoscope. 2005;115:78–80.

11. Ramadan HH, McLaughlin K, Josephson G, Rimell F, Bent J, Parikh SR. Balloon catheter sinuplasty in young children. Am J Rhinol Allergy. 2010;24:e54–6.

12. Setliff 3rd RC. The small-hole technique in endoscopic sinus surgery. Otolaryngol Clin North Am. 1997;30:341–54.

13. Lee BJ. Fungal rhinosinusitis. In: Flint P, editor. Cummings otolaryngology: head and neck surgery. 6th ed. Philadelphia: Saunders; 2015. p. 731–9.

14. Gan EC, Thamboo A, Rudmik L, Hwang PH, Ferguson BJ, Javer AR. Medical management of allergic fungal rhinosinusitis following endoscopic sinus surgery: an evidence-based review and recommendations. Int Forum Allergy Rhinol. 2014;4:702–15.

15. Laury AM, Wise SK. Chapter 7: Allergic fungal rhinosinusitis. Am J Rhinol Allergy. 2013;27 Suppl 1:S26–7.

16. Berger G, Gass S, Ophir D. The histopathology of the hypertrophic inferior turbinate. Arch Otolaryngol Head Neck Surg. 2006;132:588–94.

17. Stallman JS, Lobo JN, Som PM. The incidence of concha bullosa and its relationship to nasal septal deviation and paranasal sinus disease. AJNR Am J Neuroradiol. 2004;25:1613–8.

18. Stankiewicz JA. Primary sinus surgery. In: Flint PW, editor. Cummings otolaryngology: head and neck surgery. 6th ed. Philadelphia: Saunders; 2015. p. 752–82.

19. Bolger WE, Butzin CA, Parsons DS. Paranasal sinus bony anatomic variations and mucosal abnormalities: CT analysis for endoscopic sinus surgery. Laryngoscope. 1991;101(1 Pt 1):56–64.

20. Rice DH, Kern EB, Marple BF, Mabry RL, Friedman WH. The turbinates in nasal and sinus surgery: a consensus statement. Ear Nose Throat J. 2003;82:82–4.

21. Reitzen SD, Chung W, Shah AR. Nasal septal deviation in the pediatric and adult populations. Ear Nose Throat J. 2011;90:112–5.

22. Buyukertan M, Keklikoglu N, Kokten G. A morphometric consideration of nasal septal deviations by people with paranasal complaints; a computed tomography study. Rhinology. 2003;41:21–4.

23. Svider PF, Sheyn A, Folbe E, Sekhsaria V, Zuliani G, Eloy JA, et al. How did that get there? A population-based analysis of nasal foreign bodies. Int Forum Allergy Rhinol. 2014;4:944–9.

24. Balikci HH, Ozkul MH, Uvacin O, Yasar H, Karakas M, Gurdal M. Antrochoanal polyposis: analysis of 34 cases. Eur Arch Otorhinolaryngol. 2013;270(5):1651–4.

25. Maldonado M, Martinez A, Alobid I, Mullol J. The antrochoanal polyp. Rhinology. 2004;42:178–82.

26. Elluru RG. Congenital malformations of the nose and nasopharynx. In: Flint P, editor. Cummings otolaryngology—head and neck surgery. 6th ed. Philadelphia: Saunders; 2015. p. 2944–55.

27. Gonik NJ, Cheng J, Lesser M, Shikowitz MJ, Smith LP. Patient selection in congenital pyriform aperture stenosis repair—14 year experience and systematic review of literature. Int J Pediatr Otorhinolaryngol. 2015;79:235–9.

28. McDonald TJ, DeRemee RA. Head and neck involvement in Wegener's granulomatosis (WG). Adv Exp Med Biol. 1993;336:309–13.

29. Cannady SB, Batra PS, Koening C, Lorenz RR, Citardi MJ, Langford C, et al. Sinonasal Wegener granulomatosis: a single-institution experience with 120 cases. Laryngoscope. 2009;119:757–61.

30. Lutalo PM, D'Cruz DP. Diagnosis and classification of granulomatosis with polyangiitis (aka Wegener's granulomatosis). J Autoimmun. 2014;48–49:94–8.

31. Corrales CE, Koltai PJ. Choanal atresia: current concepts and controversies. Curr Opin Otolaryngol Head Neck Surg. 2009;17:466–70.

32. Bluestone CD, Simons J, Healy G. Pediatric otolaryngology. 5th ed. Shelton, CT: Peoples Medical Publishing House; 2014.

33. Fekete-Szabo G, Berenyi I, Gabriella K, Urban E, Nagy E. Aerobic and anaerobic bacteriology of chronic adenoid disease in children. Int J Pediatr Otorhinolaryngol. 2010;74:1217–20.

34. Shin KS, Cho SH, Kim KR, et al. The role of adenoids in pediatric rhinosinusitis. Int J Pediatr Otolaryngol. 2008;72:1643–50.

35. Brook I, Shah K. Bacteriology of adenoids and tonsils in children with recurrent adenotonsillitis. Ann Otol Rhinol Laryngol. 2001;110:844–8.

36. Brook I, Shah K, Jackson W. Microbiology of healthy and diseased adenoids. Laryngoscope. 2000;110:994–9.

37. McClay JE. Resistant bacteria in the adenoids: a preliminary report. Arch Otolaryngol Head Neck Surg. 2000;126:625–9.

38. Tuncer U, Aydogan B, Soylu L, Simsek M, Akcali C, Kucukcan A. Chronic rhinosinusitis and adenoid hypertrophy in children. Am J Otolaryngol. 2004;25:5–10.

39. Parikh SR, Coronel M, Lee JJ, Brown SM. Validation of a new grading system for endoscopic examination of adenoid hypertrophy. Otolaryngol Head Neck Surg. 2006;135:684–7.

40. Mlynarek A, Tewfik MA, Hagr A, Manoukian JJ, Schloss MD, Tewfik TL, et al. Lateral neck radiography versus direct video rhinoscopy in assessing adenoid size. J Otolaryngol. 2004;33:360–5.

41. Mossey PA, Little J. Epidemiology of oral clefts: an international perspective. In: Wyszynski DR, editor. Cleft lip and palate. From origin to treatment. New York: Oxford University Press; 2002. p. 127–44.

42. Stewart KJ, Ahmed RE, Razzell RE, Watson ACH. Altered speech following adenoidectomy: a 20 year experience. Br J Plast Surg. 2002;55:469–73.

43. Alshaikh NA, Eleftheriadou A. Juvenile nasopharyngeal angiofibroma staging: an overview. Ear Nose Throat J. 2015;94:E12–22.

44. Garofalo P, Pia F, Policarpo M, Tunesi S, Valletti PA. Juvenile nasopharyngeal angiofibroma; comparison between endoscopic and open operative approaches. J Craniofac Surg. 2015;26:918–21.

45. Healy JN, Borg MF. Paediatric nasopharyngeal rhabdomyosarcoma: a case series and literature review. J Med Imaging Radiat Oncol. 2010;54:388–94.

46. Gradoni P, Giordano D, Oretti G, Fantoni M, Ferri T. The role of surgery in children with head and neck rhabdomyosarcoma and Ewing's sarcoma. Surg Oncol. 2010;19:e103–9.

47. Gradoni P, Giordano D, Oretti G, et al. Clinical outcomes of rhabdomyosarcoma and Ewing's sarcoma of the head and neck in children. Auris Nasus Larynx. 2011;38:480–6.

48. Pakkasjarvi N, Salminen P, et al. Respiratory distress secondary to nasopharyngeal glial heterotopia. Eur J Pediatr Surg. 2008;18:117–8.

49. Husein OF, Collins M, Kang DR. Neuroglial heterotopia causing neonatal airway obstruction: presentation, management and literature review. Eur J Pediatr. 2008;167:1351–5.

50. Cohen AF, Mitsudo S, Ruben RJ. Nasopharyngeal teratoma in the neonate. Int J Pediatr Otorhinolaryngol. 1987;14:187–95.

51. Hossein A, Mohammad A. Huge teratoma of the nasopharynx. Am J Otolaryngol. 2007;28:177–9.

52. Lakhoo K. Neonatal teratomas. Early Hum Dev. 2010;86:643–7.

Oral Cavity and Oropharynx

3

Jeffrey Cheng

Oral Cavity

The oral cavity is an area that has been historically quite accessible, as illumination with a simple light may be sufficient for examination. However, visualization, magnification, and illumination with an endoscope for documentation and illustration for the 1`patient may be helpful in discussion and education. Lesions affecting the oral cavity may be of congenital, inflammatory, neoplastic, caustic, or other etiologies. Identification by the family or primary care provider may prompt consultation by the otolaryngologist. These are often benign in histological nature but may cause more concerning symptoms, such as problems with recurrent infection, respiration, and deglutition.

Oral Cavity Normal Anatomy

The oral cavity plays an integral role in dental hygiene, articulation, control of secretions, swallowing function, and other vital functions. The oral cavity is anteriorly comprised of the

J. Cheng, M.D., F.A.A.P. (✉)
Division of Pediatric Otolaryngology, Cohen
Children's Medical Center, Assistant Professor of
Otolaryngology – Head and Neck Surgery, Hofstra
North Shore – LIJ School of Medicine, 430 Lakeville
Road, New Hyde Park, NY 11042, USA
e-mail: jeffreychengmd@gmail.com

vermillion border of the lips, posteriorly by the junction of the hard and soft palate and circumvallate papilla, and laterally by the buccal mucosa (Fig. 3.1). The oral cavity is comprised of several anatomic subsites including oral tongue, floor of mouth, hard palate, buccal mucosa, retromolar trigone, and maxillary/mandibular gingival sulci. The oral cavity is primarily lined by mucosal, non-keratinizing squamous epithelium [1, 2].

Ankyloglossia

Ankyloglossia is commonly recognized in the general population as a tongue-tie and describes a congenital, persistent lingual frenulum that may restrict tongue mobility and potentially interfere with breastfeeding or speech articulation. It is fairly prevalent in the population and, depending on the reports, has a prevalence of <1–13 % [3]. This may initially be noticed around the time of birth. Newborns may be symptomatic or asymptomatic. Symptomatic newborns may present with breastfeeding challenges including maternal pain or newborn breastfeeding latch problems. Breastfeeding is a multifactorial and coordinated effort, and ankyloglossia may be a contributing factor, as the lingual frenulum may restrict full mobility of the oral tongue. Other concerns may involve potential for speech articulation and intelligibility issues when the child reaches school age, but the current evidence is

© Springer International Publishing Switzerland 2016
J. Cheng, J.P. Bent (eds.), *Endoscopic Atlas of Pediatric Otolaryngology*,
DOI 10.1007/978-3-319-29471-1_3

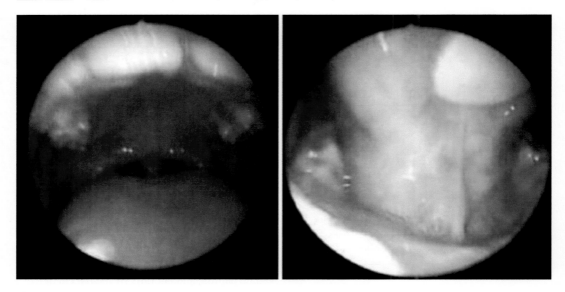

Fig. 3.1 Normal oral cavity anatomy demonstrating hard palate, tongue, buccal mucosa (*left*), and floor of mouth (*right*)

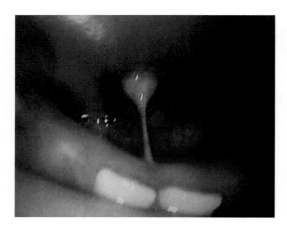

Fig. 3.2 Anterior ankyloglossia

insufficient to provide a recommendation [4]. A generalized grading system is based on the degree of attachment of the lingual frenulum to the oral tongue, with stage 1 ankyloglossia attached to the tip of the tongue, giving the tongue a classic-looking heart shape and serially decreasing by 25 % increments to stage 4 (Fig. 3.2). A posterior tongue-tie refers to restriction in tongue mobility and lack of an anterior frenulum, which is purported to arise from problematic anterior attachment of the genioglossus muscle [5]. Although the benefits of early frenotomy have yet to be elucidated,

some evidence does support improved breastfeeding experience and quality of life for appropriately selected newborns [6, 7].

Upper Lip Labial Frenum

A prominent or persistent upper labial frenulum may be present in some newborns and infants as a thick band of tissue in the midline, tethering the lingual surface of the upper lip to the mucosa of the maxillary gingiva (Fig. 3.3). The role that this may play in breastfeeding challenges, as it may restrict pursing ability of the upper lip to obtain and maintain a successful latch, is not well understood and clinical opinions differ [8].

Floor-of-Mouth Lesion

Floor-of-mouth lesions in the pediatric population are extremely uncommon. A submucosal raised floor of mouth lesion may be further evaluated by cross-sectional imaging, such as either computed tomography (CT) or magnetic resonance imaging (MRI). Congenital lesions predominate, resulting from errors in foregut embryologic development and may consist of dermoids, teratomas, or foregut

Fig. 3.3 Maxillary, upper lip labial frenulum

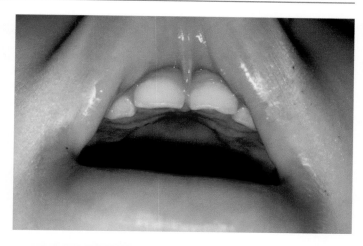

Fig. 3.4 Excision of floor-of-mouth sialolith causing right submandibular sialadenitis

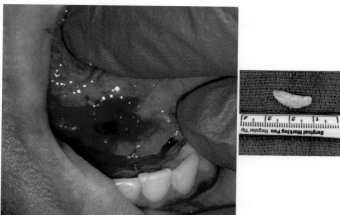

duplication cysts, which may appear as submucosal floor-of-mouth masses on examination [9]. Surgical management is primarily recommended and associated with excellent cure rates [10]. Inflammatory and infectious pathology may also affect this area, including viral, bacterial, and/or autoimmune etiologies [11]. Infections in the floor of mouth area may stem from sialoliths, which may obstruct salivary flow from the submandibular gland, resulting in submandibular gland sialadenitis. Surgical removal of the sialolith is often effective (Fig. 3.4) [12].

Oral Cavity Submucosal Tumor

Saliva production in the oral cavity originates from three, paired, major salivary glands—parotid, submandibular/submaxillary, and sublingual glands—and many minor salivary glands that are lined throughout. Their anatomic location is submucosal, and any raised submucosal lesion should raise clinical suspicion [13, 14]. The differential diagnosis for other submucosal-appearing neoplastic lesions also includes sarcomas and vascular or neural tumors, such as a schwannoma (Figs. 3.5 and 3.6) [15, 16].

Vascular Malformations

Vascular malformations are a type of vascular anomalies and may occur in the pediatric population in the oral cavity. Vascular malformations generally exist as lymphatic, venous, capillary, or arteriovenous malformations. The extent and involvement of disease can be quite variable between affected individuals; they may exist as

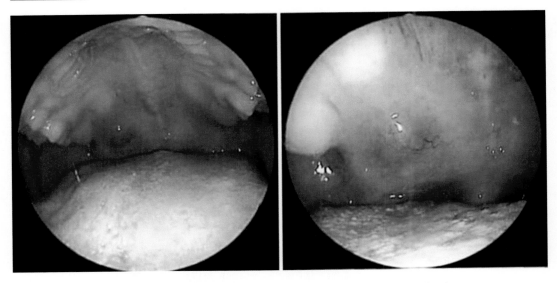

Fig. 3.5 Right hard palate submucosal schwannoma, located at the junction of hard and soft palate

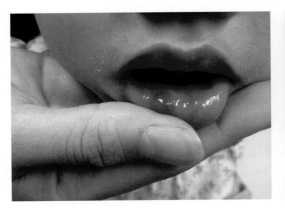

Fig. 3.6 Lower lip submucosal mucus retention cyst

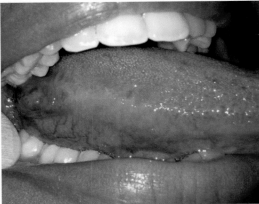

Fig. 3.7 Lymphatic malformation, right lateral oral tongue

well-localized, solitary lesions to diffusely spread out submucosal involvement (Fig. 3.7). Generally, management decisions are individualized and based on the child's symptoms and expected natural clinical history of disease. Treatment may involve any combination of watchful waiting or expectant management, sclerotherapy, surgical resection, and/or immunomodulatory medications [17].

Oral Cavity Mucosal Lesion or Ulceration

The mucosal lining of the oral cavity may develop focal or multifocal ulcers in response to inflammatory, caustic/iatrogenic, neoplastic, or infectious etiologies (Fig. 3.8). Caustic ingestions are becoming more prevalent with changes in industry packaging for different household products, such as laundry detergent [18]. Clinical decision making in management of children presenting with this problem may range from active intervention to observation and supportive management [19].

Oropharynx

The oropharynx is subdivided into four main areas: soft palate, posterior pharyngeal wall, palatine tonsils, and base of tongue (Fig. 3.9). Children are

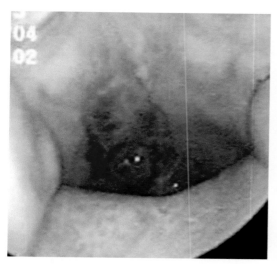

Fig. 3.8 Oral cavity mucosal lesion with right hard and soft palate involvement, pathology consistent with infantile hemangioma (GLUT-1 immunohistochemistry positive)

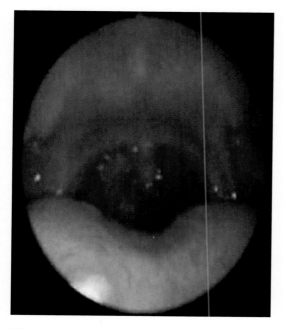

Fig. 3.9 Oropharynx normal anatomy

commonly affected by hypertrophic or infectious/inflammatory disorders of this area. The oropharynx plays an integral role in speech and swallowing. The soft palate plays an important functional role in speech production, as phonetics involving plosives depend on the soft palate to create adequate sphincter control to prevent leakage of air into the

nasopharynx. Furthermore, during swallowing, the soft palate also prevents reflux of oral intake into the nasopharynx [20]. The base of tongue, palatine tonsils, and posterior pharyngeal wall may all be affected by hypertrophy, neoplastic, inflammatory, iatrogenic, and other pathologies, but most commonly in children contributes to sleep-disordered breathing/sleep apnea. Infections of the deep neck spaces can also extend to this area, and other pathologies in this area may cause issues with swallowing or respiration.

Tonsil Hypertrophy

The palatine tonsils consist of lymphoid tissue that may undergo hypertrophic growth starting at a young age. This may result in sleep-disordered breathing symptoms in children, which commonly prompt evaluation by the otolaryngologist. Tonsil hypertrophy is graded from 1+ to 4+. The tonsil-size grading system increases by increments of 25 %, with 1+ tonsil hypertrophy being <25 % obstruction of the oropharynx, 2+ tonsil hypertrophy obstructing 26–50 %, 3+ tonsil hypertrophy obstructing 51–75 %, and 4+ tonsil hypertrophy obstructing 76–100 % of the oropharynx (Fig. 3.10) [21]. This is an extremely common problem encountered by otolaryngologists and pediatricians. Clinical assessment is directed at determining the clinical severity of the problem and the role of medical and/or surgical intervention, as well as discussing with the family our understanding of the natural clinical history of the problem. At this time, our current understanding of tonsil hypertrophy and hyperplasia and the natural history is that there is a period of lymphoid growth within the palatine tonsils during childhood, but no well-elucidated role of the palatine tonsils has been elucidated in the literature [22].

Acute Tonsillitis and Peritonsillar Cellulitis/Abscess

Acute infections of the palatine tonsils usually present with fever, throat pain, and difficulty swallowing. These are characterized on physical

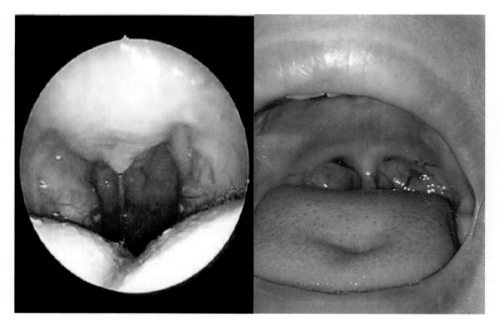

Fig. 3.10 Palatine tonsil hypertrophy, 2+ (*left*) and 3+ (*right*)

examination by erythema, induration, and swelling. Exudate and/or purulence may also be common. If bacterial in origin, antibiotics may be utilized for treatment, but the etiology may also be viral, stemming from Epstein-Barr virus (EBV), cytomegalovirus (CMV), or others. Treatment may be supportive in nature and/or directed at the underlying etiology [23, 24].

Infection may spread from the palatine tonsillar tissue laterally into a potential space located between the tonsil and the tonsillar capsule. Characteristic features include a "hot-potato" voice, unilateral throat or neck pain, difficulty controlling secretions, dysphagia, and odynophagia. Physical examination findings may include fever, trismus, uvular deviation, or peritonsillar erythema, and induration (Fig. 3.11) [25]. In some cases, a suppurative infection may develop in the peritonsillar space and become a peritonsillar abscess, which may be managed medically with antibiotics or operative incision and drainage or needle aspiration [26]. Children who are younger, have fewer episodes of acute tonsil infections, and have smaller peritonsillar abscess collections may be more successfully treated with nonoperative management [27].

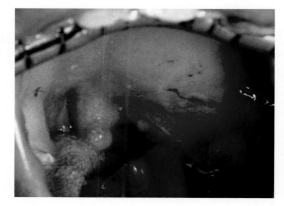

Fig. 3.11 Left peritonsillar abscess

Squamous Papilloma

Oropharyngeal papillomas in children are relatively uncommon but generally have a characteristic exophytic, "mushroom-like" appearance on physical examination (Fig. 3.12). Presenting symptoms may include no complaints, dysphagia, bleeding, or globus sensation, and histologically these lesions are typically benign in appearance [28]. Symptomatic or clinically concerning lesions are usually treated with surgical excision [29].

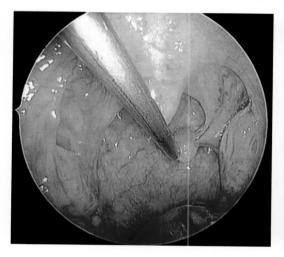

Fig. 3.12 Oropharyngeal papilloma originating from left palatopharyngeal muscle mucosa

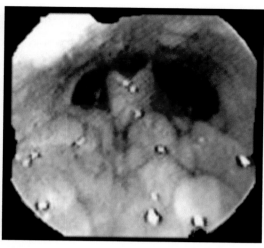

Fig. 3.14 Lingual tonsil hypertrophy

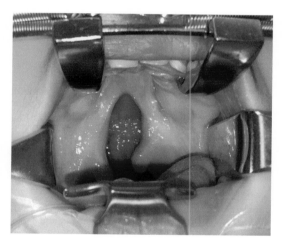

Fig. 3.13 Cleft palate

morphogenetic sequence and cascade of events, along with rapid proliferative expansion, guide the development of the facial structures early in utero. Thus, the facial structures are highly susceptible to environmental and genetic factors. The embryo's head and facial structures derive from the growth of five primitive tissue lobes: one from the fronto-nasal prominence, two from the maxillary promi-nence, and two from the mandibular prominence. If any of these tissues fail to fuse, a cleft may develop. Cleft palates are generally repaired oper-atively, as they cause cosmetic and functional problems with speech and feeding, and postopera-tively if there is incompetence of the velopharynx, this may result in impaired speech intelligibility and articulation [30].

Cleft Palate

Nonunion of the hard and/or the soft palate is one of the most commonly occurring congenital anomalies (Fig. 3.13). It may occur in an isolated setting or in association with other congenital genetic syndromes or congenital anomalies. When associated with syndromic cases, genetic factors may be identified, but in the more common iso-lated cases, environmental, developmental, and other genetic factors may be involved but at this time are incompletely understood. A complex

Lingual Tonsil Hypertrophy

Lymphoid tissue is located throughout Waldeyer's ring in the oropharynx, which includes areas in the base of tongue. Lingual tonsil hypertrophy may be implicated in persistent obstructive sleep apnea (OSA) in children despite adenotonsillec-tomy (Fig. 3.14) [31]. The diagnosis can be made with office endoscopy, operative sleep endoscopy, CT, and/or MRI. Lingual tonsillectomy in selected cases may be safe and effective for man-agement [32].

References

1. Huber MA, Tantiwongkosi B. Oral and oropharyngeal cancer. Med Clin North Am. 2014;98(6):1299–321.
2. Kosko JR, Moser JD, Erhart N, Tunkel DE. Differential diagnosis of dysphagia in children. Otolaryngol Clin North Am. 1998;31(3):435–51.
3. Brookes A, Bowley DM. Tongue tie: the evidence for frenotomy. Early Hum Dev. 2014;90(11):765–8.
4. Chinnadurai S, Francis DO, Epstein RA, Morad A, Kohanim S, McPheeters M. Treatment of ankyloglossia for reasons other than breastfeeding: a systematic review. Pediatrics. 2015;135(6):e1467–74.
5. Hong P, Lago D, Seargeant J, Pellman L, Magit AE, Pransky SM. Defining ankyloglossia: a case series of anterior and posterior tongue ties. Int J Pediatr Otorhinolaryngol. 2010;74(9):1003–6.
6. Francis DO, Krishnaswami S, McPheeters M. Treatment of ankyloglossia and breastfeeding outcomes: a systematic review. Pediatrics. 2015;135(6):e1458–66.
7. Francis DO, Chinnadurai S, Morad A, Epstein RA, Kohanim S, Krishnaswami S, et al. Treatments for ankyloglossia and ankyloglossia with concomitant lip-tie [Internet]. Rockville, MD: Agency for Healthcare Research and Quality (US); 2015 May. Report No.: 15-EHC011-EF.
8. Pransky SM, Lago D, Hong P. Breastfeeding difficulties and oral cavity anomalies: the influence of posterior ankyloglossia and upper-lip ties. Int J Pediatr Otorhinolaryngol. 2015;79(10):1714–7.
9. Gaddikeri S, Vattoth S, Gaddikeri RS, Stuart R, Harrison K, Young D, et al. Congenital cystic neck masses: embryology and imaging appearances, with clinicopathological correlation. Curr Probl Diagn Radiol. 2014;43(2):55–67.
10. Makos C, Noussios G, Peios M, Gougousis S, Chouridis P. Dermoid cysts of the floor of the mouth: two case reports. Case Rep Med. 2011;2011:362170.
11. Francis CL, Larsen CG. Pediatric sialadenitis. Otolaryngol Clin North Am. 2014;47(5):763–78.
12. Waseem Z, Forte V. An unusual case of bilateral submandibular sialolithiasis in a young female patient. Int J Pediatr Otorhinolaryngol. 2005;69(5):691–4.
13. Werther PL, Alawi F, Lindemeyer RG. Mucoepidermoid carcinoma of the palate in adolescence. J Dent Child (Chic). 2015;82(1):57–61.
14. Varan A, Akyuz C, Atas E, Yücel T, Aydın B, Yalçın B, et al. Salivary gland tumors in children: a retrospective clinical review. Pediatr Hematol Oncol. 2014;31(8):681–6.
15. Satish V, Bhat M, Maganur PC, Shah P, Biradar V. Capillary hemangioma in maxillary anterior region: a case report. Int J Clin Pediatr Dent. 2014;7(2):144–7.
16. Shrutha SP, Vinit GB. Rhabdomyosarcoma in a pediatric patient: a rare case report. Contemp Clin Dent. 2015;6(1):113–5.
17. Hoff SR, Rastatter JC, Richter GT. Head and neck vascular lesions. Otolaryngol Clin North Am. 2015;48(1):29–45.
18. Beuhler MC, Gala PK, Wolfe HA, Meaney PA, Henretig FM. Laundry detergent "pod" ingestions: a case series and discussion of recent literature. Pediatr Emerg Care. 2013;29(6):743–7.
19. Karjoo M. Caustic ingestion and foreign bodies in the gastrointestinal system. Curr Opin Pediatr. 1998;10(5):516–22.
20. Jaffer NM, Ng E, Au FW, Steele CM. Fluoroscopic evaluation of oropharyngeal dysphagia: anatomic, technical, and common etiologic factors. AJR Am J Roentgenol. 2015;204(1):49–58.
21. Trosman I. Childhood obstructive sleep apnea syndrome: a review of the 2012 American Academy of Pediatrics guidelines. Pediatr Ann. 2013;42(10):195–9.
22. Baugh RF, Archer SM, Mitchell RB, Rosenfeld RM, Amin R, Burns JJ, et al. Clinical practice guideline: tonsillectomy in children. Otolaryngol Head Neck Surg. 2011;144(1 Suppl):S1–30.
23. Baltimore RS. Re-evaluation of antibiotic treatment of streptococcal pharyngitis. Curr Opin Pediatr. 2010;22(1):77–82.
24. Sih TM, Bricks LF. Optimizing the management of the main acute infections in pediatric ORL: tonsillitis, sinusitis, otitis media. Braz J Otorhinolaryngol. 2008;74(5):755–62.
25. Hsiao HJ, Huang YC, Hsia SH, Wu CT, Lin JJ. Clinical features of peritonsillar abscess in children. Pediatr Neonatol. 2012;53(6):366–70.
26. Qureshi H, Ference E, Novis S, Pritchett CV, Smith SS, Schroeder JW. Trends in the management of pediatric peritonsillar abscess infections in the U.S., 2000–2009. Int J Pediatr Otorhinolaryngol. 2015;79(4):527–31.
27. Kim DK, Lee JW, Na YS, Kim MJ, Lee JH, Park CH. Clinical factor for successful nonsurgical treatment of pediatric peritonsillar abscess. Laryngoscope. 2015;125(11):2608–11.
28. Devi RS, Rajsekhar B, Srinivas GV, Moon NJ. Unusual length of pedicle: pedunculated squamous papilloma of uvula causing unusual Dysphagia of long duration in a child of 10 years. Case Rep Dent. 2014;2014:313506.
29. Crockett DM, Healy GB, McGill TJ, Friedman EM. Benign lesions of the nose, oral cavity, and oropharynx in children: excision by carbon dioxide laser. Ann Otol Rhinol Laryngol. 1985;94(5 Pt 1):489–93.
30. Gart MS, Gosain AK. Surgical management of velopharyngeal insufficiency. Clin Plast Surg. 2014;41(2):253–70.
31. Friedman NR, Prager JD, Ruiz AG, Kezirian EJ. A pediatric grading scale for lingual tonsil hypertrophy. Otolaryngol Head Neck Surg. 2015 Aug 25. pii: 0194599815601403 (Epub ahead of print).
32. Abdel-Aziz M, Ibrahim N, Ahmed A, El-Hamamsy M, Abdel-Khalik MI, El-Hoshy H. Lingual tonsils hypertrophy; a cause of obstructive sleep apnea in children after adenotonsillectomy: operative problems and management. Int J Pediatr Otorhinolaryngol. 2011;75(9):1127–31.

Airway and Aerodigestive Tract

4

Jeffrey Cheng and Lee P. Smith

Supraglottis

The supraglottis has several anatomic subsites: vallecula, epiglottis, arytenoids, and false vocal folds. Primary lesions of the supraglottis in pediatric patients are most commonly congenital in origin but may also be infectious or iatrogenic. The focus in evaluation and management of these pathologies should be on their effect on feeding, weight gain, growth, and development. Lesions at any level of the pediatric airway and aerodigestive tract can contribute to failure to thrive, feeding intolerance, or growth and development impediments, but pathology at this level of the pediatric airway is more commonly encountered in newborns, infants, and very young children (Fig. 4.1).

Laryngomalacia

Laryngomalacia is the most common cause of stridor in infants. Characteristic endoscopy findings include shortened aryepiglottic folds and an omega-shaped epiglottis and dynamic features of arytenoid and/or epiglottic prolapse, which obstruct the view of the glottis airway (Fig. 4.2). The stridor results from collapse of the supraglottic tissues into the glottic inlet, resulting in turbulent airflow. In most instances, expectant management may be advised, as the natural clinical history and evolution usually result in self-resolution. Evaluation with office-based flexible endoscopy is helpful to make the diagnosis and exclude other airway pathology. In some cases, laryngomalacia may result in failure to thrive, feeding difficulties, acute life-threatening events, or persistent exertional stridor or sleep apnea after 18 months of age. Surgical intervention with supraglottoplasty should be considered and is usually very effective for these more significant cases (Fig. 4.3). Proper patient selection and identification of patients with severe symptoms are paramount for providing successful outcomes [1–3].

Vascular Malformations

Venous and lymphatic malformations are types of vascular anomalies consisting of dilated venous and/or lymphatic channels, which may affect any

J. Cheng, M.D., F.A.A.P. (✉) • L.P. Smith, M.D.
Division of Pediatric Otolaryngology,
Cohen Children's Medical Center, Assistant Professor of Otolaryngology – Head and Neck Surgery, Hofstra North Shore – LIJ School of Medicine, 430 Lakeville Road, New Hyde Park, NY 11042, USA
e-mail: jeffreychengmd@gmail.com; lsmith8@nshs.edu

© Springer International Publishing Switzerland 2016
J. Cheng, J.P. Bent (eds.), *Endoscopic Atlas of Pediatric Otolaryngology*,
DOI 10.1007/978-3-319-29471-1_4

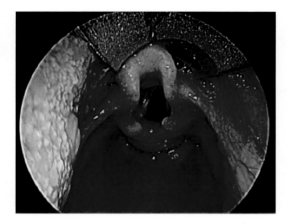

Fig. 4.1 Normal supraglottis

site within the head and neck (Fig. 4.4). These lesions are generally present at birth and grow proportionately with the child. When in the aerodigestive tract, over time these may begin to exert and exhibit a mass effect, resulting in dysphagia, dysphonia, respiratory symptoms, or pain (Fig. 4.5). Management focuses on understanding the natural history and clinical evolution as well as severity of symptoms. These often become symptomatic sometime in the patient's life. Treatment options include medical, surgical, and/or interventional radiology-based procedures, depending on the extent and type of lesion. Various endoscopic and open surgical techniques have been described for management (Fig. 4.6) [4–9].

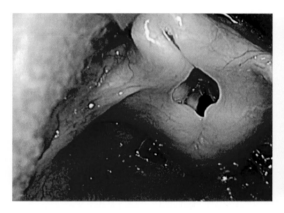

Fig. 4.2 Laryngomalacia, combination type 1 (prolapsing arytenoids) and 2 (shortened aryepiglottic folds)

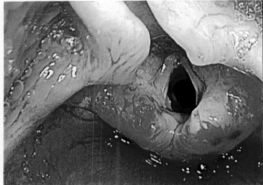

Fig. 4.3 Postoperative result after supraglottoplasty— cold steel surgical technique

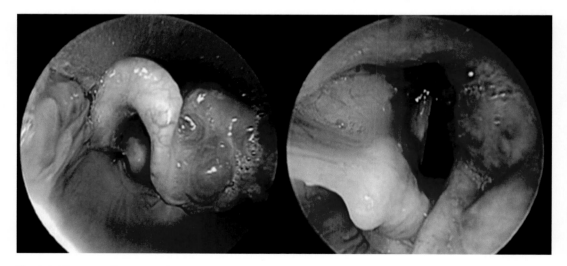

Fig. 4.4 Venous malformation of supraglottis

Epiglottitis/Supraglottitis

Epiglottitis or supraglottitis historically was predominantly the result of infectious etiologies (Fig. 4.7). Classically, these children present in extremis with severe odynophagia, fevers, inability to tolerate secretions or lie supine, and toxic appearance. With the advent of widespread vaccination for *Haemophilus influenzae*, the incidence has dramatically decreased. Primary treatment focuses on airway management and medical management of the infection [10–12].

Vallecular Cyst

Vallecular cysts are rare causes of stridor in infants that may present similarly to laryngomalacia (Figs. 4.8 and 4.9). Office-based endoscopy is useful to distinguish these two entities; how-

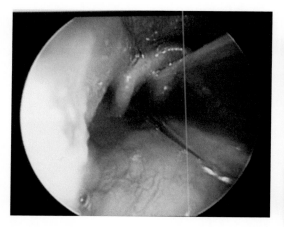

Fig. 4.5 Lymphatic malformation presenting with acute hemorrhage involving the posterior pharyngeal wall and supraglottic larynx

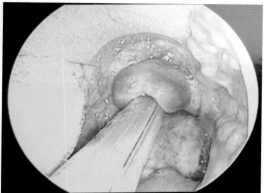

Fig. 4.7 Indurated and edematous epiglottis, illustrating epiglottis

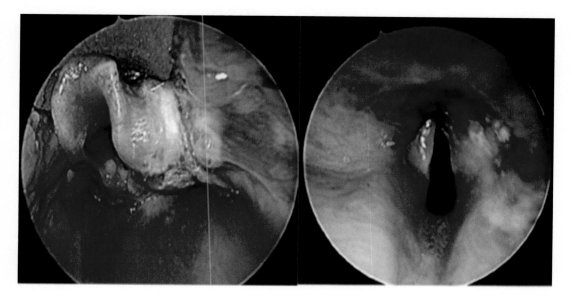

Fig. 4.6 Postoperative results after potassium titanyl phosphate (KTP) laser ablation of supraglottic venous malformation

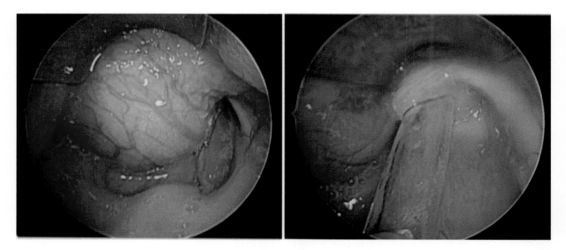

Fig. 4.8 Vallecular cyst, primarily left sided and nearly obstructive

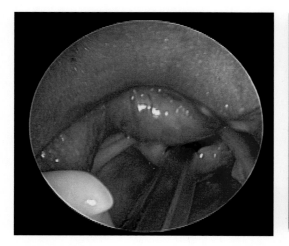

Fig. 4.9 Vallecular cyst

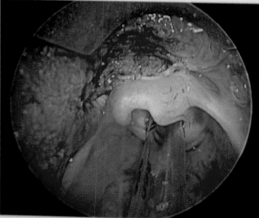

Fig. 4.10 Immediate postoperative result after cold steel dissection and removal of vallecular cyst

ever, given the technical challenges of fiber-optic laryngoscopy in newborns and young infants, it may be easy to confuse the findings on fiber-optic endoscopy with laryngomalacia. Surgical excision or marsupialization is the treatment of choice, as these infants are often symptomatic. Successful endoscopic treatment with CO_2 laser, radiofrequency ablation, and cold dissection have all been described (Fig. 4.10) [13–15]. These lesions may also resemble lingual thyroid tissue or neoplasms.

Glottis

Understanding the structure and function of the vocal cords is essential in the evaluation and management of glottic pathology (Figs. 4.11 and 4.12). At birth, many different organ systems are immature and undergo significant histologic and morphologic changes. The classic model of the mature vocal cord, from superficial to deep, includes a composition of three distinct layers: a

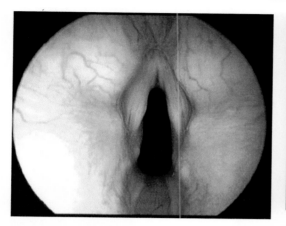

Fig. 4.11 Normal glottis

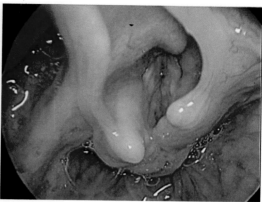

Fig. 4.13 Laryngeal stenosis in a premature newborn male with prolonged intubation

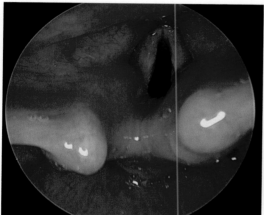

Fig. 4.12 Normal glottis

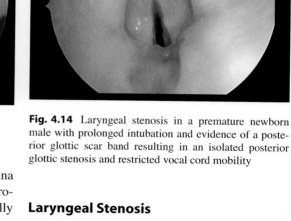

Fig. 4.14 Laryngeal stenosis in a premature newborn male with prolonged intubation and evidence of a posterior glottic scar band resulting in an isolated posterior glottic stenosis and restricted vocal cord mobility

nonkeratinizing stratified squamous layer, lamina propria, and the vocalis muscle. The lamina propria is further composed of three histologically separate layers—superficial, middle, and deep—which are believed to play a significant role in the fibrovascular and viscoelastic properties of the vocal folds. The middle and deep layers of the lamina propria are intimately related and make up the vocal ligament, which in neonates comprises approximately half the length of the vocal cord, as opposed to one-third the length of the vocal cord in adults [16].

Laryngeal Stenosis

Prolonged intubation in newborns can lead to laryngeal stenosis, which at the glottic level is primarily secondary to posterior glottic stenosis (Figs. 4.13, 4.14, and 4.15). Congenital laryngeal atresia presents as a critical airway obstruction and is a rare cause of respiratory distress in newborns. This may be found in the presence of a tracheoesophageal fistula, esophageal atresia, encephalocele, or

Fig. 4.15 Complex
laryngeal stenosis with
arytenoid scarring

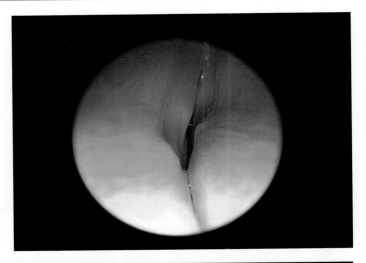

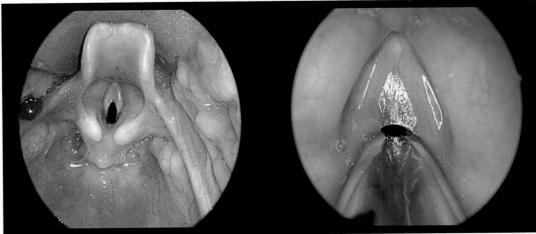

Fig. 4.16 Anterior glottic web in an infant born with a thin congenital anterior glottic web

congenital high airway obstructive syndrome (CHAOS) [17]. In some cases, this pathology can be identified antenatally because of fetal hydrops. With appropriate planning the airway can be secured at the time of delivery using an ex utero intrapartum treatment (EXIT) procedure. In some cases, other associated airway abnormalities, such as tracheal agenesis, may cause this congenital anomaly to be incompatible with life [18–21].

Anterior Glottic Web

Anterior glottic webs may be of congenital or acquired origin (Fig. 4.16). Acquired anterior glottic webs are more commonly found in adults and may be treated endoscopically or open, with or

without the placement of a keel to prevent reformation of the synechiae [22–24]. Congenital anterior glottic webs are much less common and may present in the newborn period with dysphonia, stridor, or respiratory distress. Management may include watchful waiting, endoscopic lysis with or without keel placement, open airway reconstruction, or tracheotomy [25–27]. Fluorescence in situ hybridization (FISH) testing may be warranted to investigate for 22q11 deletion syndrome [28].

Laryngeal Papilloma

Laryngeal papilloma in children is the result of human papilloma virus (HPV) infection, usually serotypes 6 and 11 (Fig. 4.17). The virus affects

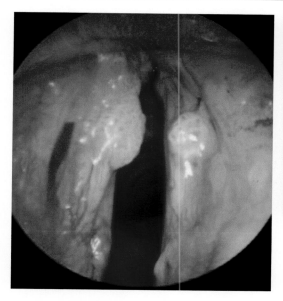

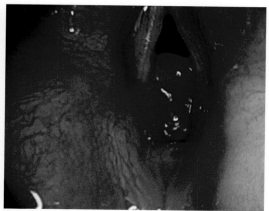

Fig. 4.18 Post-intubation vocal process granuloma

Fig. 4.17 Glottic papillomatosis

the nonkeratinizing squamous epithelium of the larynx and may over time spread distally into the tracheobronchial tree. Most commonly, these patients present with dysphonia but in some cases they may present with stridor and/or respiratory distress, as the extent of disease involvement may cause critical airway obstruction. Treatment is generally focused on debulking the disease with microlaryngeal surgical techniques. Children with persistent and recurrent diffuse disease may benefit from other adjuvant therapies. Younger patients, less than 3 years of age, and those with HPV-11 may be more prone to more severe disease, as they have been found to have greater extent of disease burden at the time of endoscopic debridement, more frequent operative treatments, and increased rates of adjuvant therapy [29]. The role of HPV vaccination for the prevention or management of this disease is unknown at this time.

Vocal Fold Granuloma

Vocal fold granulomas are uncommonly encountered but may be the result of traumatic intubation, gastroesophageal reflux disease (GERD), or contact (Fig. 4.18). In newborns, infants, and children, this generally is the result of traumatic endotracheal intubation, which results in the

development of significant inflammation and granulation tissue formation. These lesions are located at the vocal process, which is where the vocal ligament posteriorly attaches to the base of the arytenoid, but may also be present anteriorly [30]. The presentation often depends on the age of the child and may include respiratory distress, stridor, or hoarseness [31]. The diagnosis can be made with flexible laryngoscopy and/or rigid microlaryngoscopy. These appear as an exophytic lesion, usually unilaterally. Traumatic vocal fold granulomas in symptomatic patients are usually responsive to microlaryngeal excision.

Elevated True Vocal Fold Lesions

Elevated true vocal fold lesions may be a common etiology for dysphonia in children. The lesions may originate from the mucosal, nonkeratinizing, squamous epithelium or the submucosal space. The differential diagnosis may include, but not limited to, vocal cord nodule, submucosal cyst, pseudocyst, and hemorrhagic or non-hemorrhagic polyp (Fig. 4.19). They may cause significant voice disability, especially functional [32].

Subglottis

The cricoid cartilage is at the level of the subglottis and is the only complete ring in the pediatric airway (Fig. 4.20). Because of its fixed diameter and relatively smaller radius and dimension than the adult cricoid cartilage, this area of the pediatric airway is especially sensitive to inflammatory, infectious, and iatrogenic pathology.

Subglottic Stenosis

The etiology of subglottic stenosis may be congenital or acquired. Acquired subglottic stenosis in newborns and infants is most commonly a complication related to endotracheal intubation (Fig. 4.21). Severity of the disease usually dictates the management strategy. Endoscopic balloon dilation is becoming more established as a highly effective strategy for the management of children with subglottic stenosis (Figs. 4.22 and 4.23). Balloon dilation can be used as a primary mode of treatment or as an adjunct to open airway reconstruction [33, 34]. Other treatment options include tracheostomy and open laryngotracheal reconstruction [35–39].

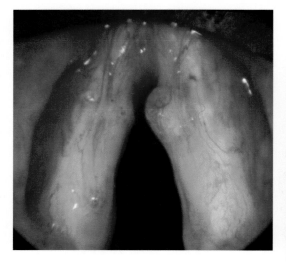

Fig. 4.19 Right true vocal fold submucosal cyst with reactive left true vocal fold nodule

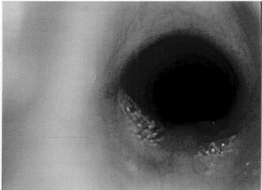

Fig. 4.20 Normal subglottis

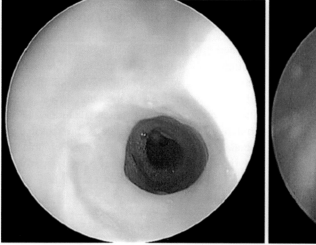

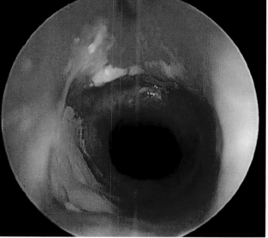

Fig. 4.21 Grade 2 thin subglottic stenosis resulting from difficult intubation in full-term, 3-month-old female (*left*). Immediate result after endoscopy balloon dilation (*right*)

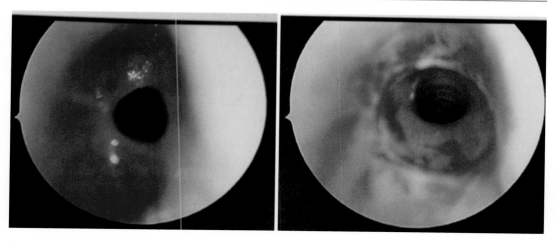

Fig. 4.22 Premature infant with prolonged intubation and postextubation stridor and positive pressure requirement before (*left*) and after (*right*) endoscopic balloon dilation

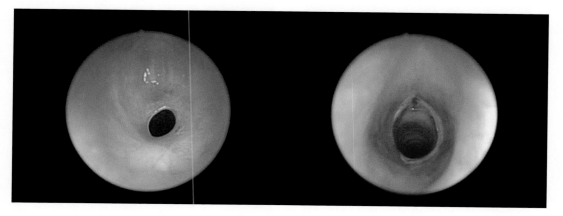

Fig. 4.23 Young child with a history of endotracheal intubation and postextubation stridor. Grade 3 isolated subglottic stenosis consisting of a thin web before (*left*) and after (*right*) endoscopic lysis with cold knife technique and balloon dilation

Subglottic Cysts

Subglottic cysts often result after endotracheal intubation and can occur following even short periods of intubation (Fig. 4.24). Laryngoscopy and bronchoscopy are important in establishing the diagnosis. These are relatively uncommon causes of airway obstruction and may be asymptomatic. Treatment is indicated for symptomatic cysts, which can be single or multiple (Figs. 4.25 and 4.26). Endoscopic marsupialization is the favored management strategy in symptomatic cases and can be accomplished with any number or combination of microlaryngeal instruments and techniques, including powered microdebridement, electrodessication, CO_2 laser, or cold steel. Endoscopic management is often successful and may result in immediate resolution of symptoms even for those patients with critical airway obstruction [40–43].

Subglottic Hemangioma

Recurrent croup-like symptoms in infants less than 6 months of age who have no history of endotracheal intubation should raise clinical suspicion for subglottic hemangioma (Figs. 4.27 and 4.28).

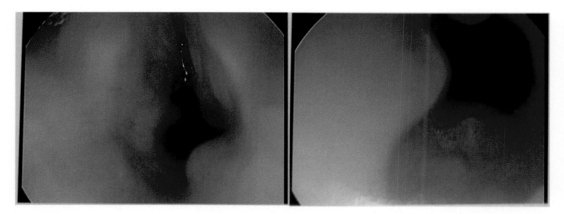

Fig. 4.24 Multiple subglottic cysts

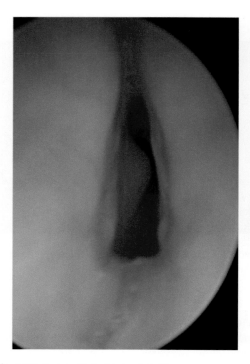

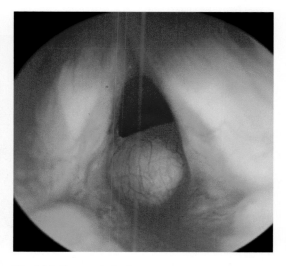

Fig. 4.26 Large subglottic cyst

Fig. 4.25 Isolated left-sided subglottic cyst

Historically, several different management strategies have been discussed and advocated, including intralesional and/or systemic corticosteroids, laser resection, open surgical excision, and tracheotomy. Each is associated with its shortcomings and risks. Recently, the management paradigm has shifted toward propranolol therapy as the primary mainstay of treatment, reserving other treatment modalities for propranolol nonresponders or those

infants who cannot tolerate the medication. Propranolol has demonstrated significant clinical efficacy with well-tolerated side effects and has become a favored treatment option [44–47].

Postintubation Subglottic Trauma

Endotracheal intubation, even for a short duration, may cause acute inflammatory changes secondary to the foreign body instrumentation and applied pressure to the mucosal surface of the subglottis. Clinical symptoms may vary from none to stridor with or without respiratory decompensation.

Endoscopic features may include varying degrees if mucosal ulceration and subglottic edema (Fig. 4.29). After extubation, these endoscopic findings can be temporary with full recovery and resolution of the mucosal ulceration and inflammation, or chronic and permanent scar formation may ensue, resulting in subglottic stenosis [48].

Croup

Croup is by far the most common cause of stridor in children and is caused by a viral infection, classically involving the parainfluenza virus.

Clinically, the entity is characterized by upper respiratory viral symptoms, fever, barky cough, and noisy breathing. Generally, it is self-limited in its natural clinical history and may be managed with supportive therapy and reassurance. In other cases, however, in some children, such as those with underlying medical and respiratory comorbidities, the clinical presentation and severity of disease may cause more respiratory symptoms necessitating further therapy [49, 50]. One of the main objectives of medical management is to avoid endotracheal intubation, as the inflammatory process that affects the subglottis in this circumstance may cause significant, continued, and deleterious scarring (Fig 4.30). The endotracheal tube adds an additional nidus for

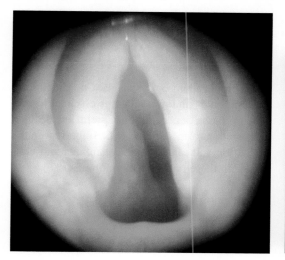

Fig. 4.27 Subglottic hemangioma, classic based left posterolaterally

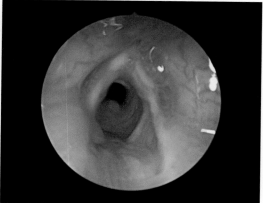

Fig. 4.29 Diffuse subglottic ulceration secondary to prolonged endotracheal intubation

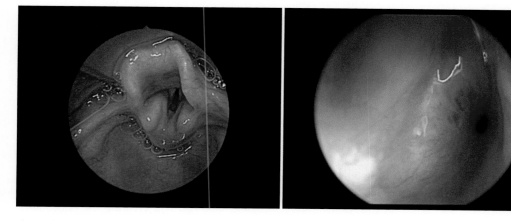

Fig. 4.28 Subglottic hemangioma, untreated. Subglottic fullness (*left*) and, upon closer inspection, significant narrowing of subglottic lumen (*right*)

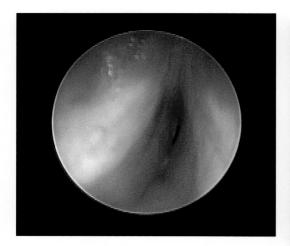

Fig. 4.30 Severe croup, subglottic circumferential mucosal, and submucosal edema

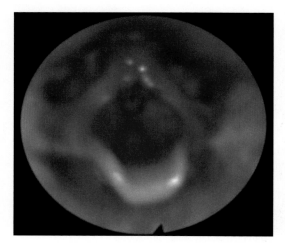

Fig. 4.31 Normal hypopharynx as seen by fiber-optic examination

inflammation and may cause prolonged hospitalization and recovery. However, in some circumstances, this may be unavoidable in the child presenting in extremis [51].

Hypopharynx

The hypopharynx is anatomically subdivided into three areas: left and right pyriform sinuses, postcricoid area, and posterior pharyngeal wall (Figs. 4.31 and 4.32). In infants and children, congenital anomalies often lead to recurrent infec-

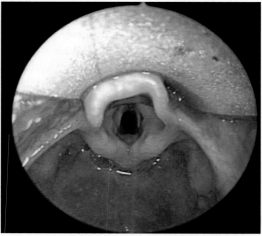

Fig. 4.32 Normal hypopharynx as seen by direct laryngoscopy and magnified with optical endoscope

tious complications or dysphagia. Coordination of the food bolus and oral intake is essential to prevent aspiration or penetration. Careful and detailed examination of this area may be important in the evaluation and management of infants and children with these presenting symptoms.

Laryngeal Cleft

Considerable evidence is mounting that type 1 laryngeal clefts and normal anatomy with functional incompetence of the interarytenoid area may be contributing to dysphagia, aspiration, and recurrent pneumonia in some children (Fig. 4.33). Endoscopic repair of laryngeal clefts and/ or injection augmentation of this area have been demonstrated to improve chronic aspiration (Figs. 4.34 and 4.35) [52, 53]. More extensive laryngeal clefts, such as types 2 and 3, are often more difficult to manage. Type 4 laryngeal clefts are nearly all incompatible with life.

Postcricoid Venous Plexus

Vascular engorgement creating the appearance of a mass in the postcricoid area in children may often be mistaken for a vascular anomaly

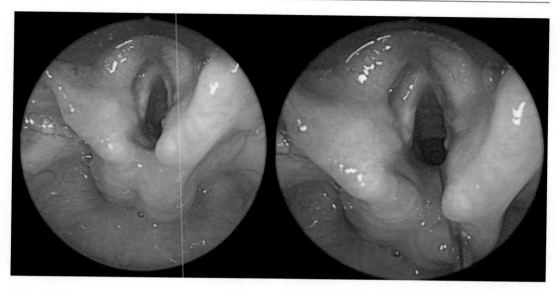

Fig. 4.33 Type 1 laryngeal cleft (*left*). Palpation of the interarytenoid area is often required to fully elucidate whether or not a cleft is present (*right*)

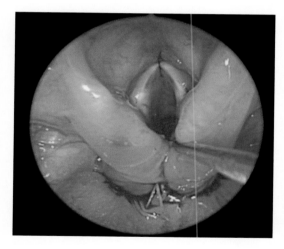

Fig. 4.34 Type 1 laryngeal cleft following endoscopic repair

Pyriform Sinus Fistula

Recurrent deep-space neck infections should raise clinical suspicion for an underlying branchial or congenital anomaly in children. Some controversy exists over the proper terminology for third and/or fourth branchial anomalies, but these lesions often present as recurrent neck infections or suppurative thyroiditis. An overwhelming majority of these lesions affect the left side (Fig. 4.37). Optimal management is often debated, but strategies include excision of the fistula tract in combination with ipsilateral hemithyroidectomy or endoscopic cauterization/de-epithelialization of the pyriform sinus tract [55–58].

or tumor (Fig. 4.36). Anatomic studies have elucidated an extensive venous plexus in this anatomic area of the larynx. With crying or other Valsalva-type maneuvers, this area may fill and create the illusion of a mass during endoscopic examination. This may be a normal physiologic finding and has been postulated to serve as a protective barrier for esophageal regurgitation [54].

Trachea

The normal shape of the tracheal rings resembles a horseshoe or "U" shape, as the normal anatomy consists of the incomplete tracheal rings with a posterior membranous wall that is shared with the esophagus (Figs. 4.38 and 4.39). Any significant change to the composition of this anatomy may result in stridor or airway challenges.

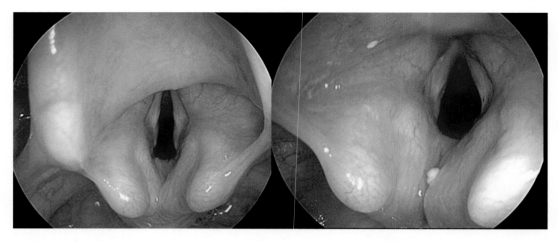

Fig. 4.35 Type 1 laryngeal cleft before and after injection augmentation of the interarytenoid area

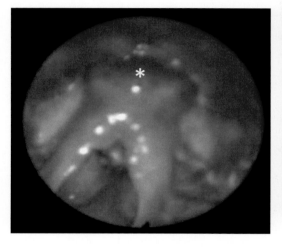

Fig. 4.36 Postcricoid venous plexus (*asterisk*) as seen by flexible fiber-optic exam

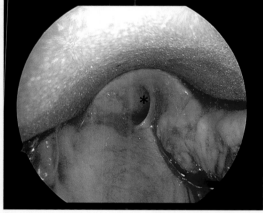

Fig. 4.37 Pyriform sinus fistula, third/fourth branchial anomaly. Direct laryngoscopy of the left pyriform sinus and fistula opening (*asterisk*)

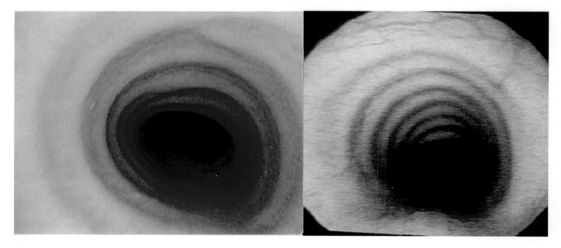

Fig. 4.38 Normal trachea

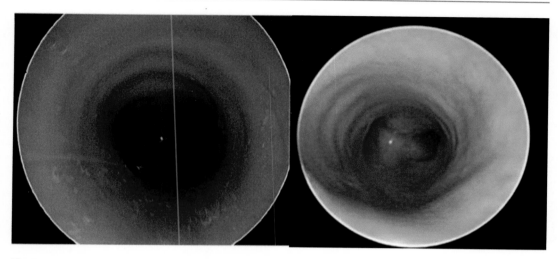

Fig. 4.39 Normal carina and right and left mainstem bronchi

Airway Foreign Body

Oral exploration by developing young infants and children is a natural way that they get to interact with their environment. There is also not yet dentition to support fully processing some foods without them becoming potentially lodged in the airway if aspirated. In combination, this may lead to foreign body aspiration in the pediatric population and can cause significant morbidity and potential mortality. Detailed history and physical examination are crucial in establishing the diagnosis. Radiographs and other ancillary tests may be used in combination with history and physical examination to determine whether operative bronchoscopy is indicated for further evaluation and treatment. Aspirated-food foreign bodies are the most commonly encountered ones (Figs. 4.40 and 4.41). Rigid bronchoscopy under general anesthesia is the preferred management strategy if an aspirated foreign body is suspected (Fig. 4.42) [59–63].

Tracheal Stenosis

The cricoid cartilage is normally the only complete ring in the airway. Stenosis of the trachea may result from congenital or acquired etiologies (Fig. 4.43). Complete tracheal rings are a type of congenital tracheal stenosis (Fig. 4.44). Children with complete tracheal rings may present with

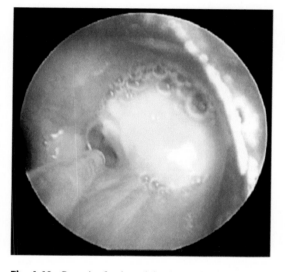

Fig. 4.40 Organic, food particle airway foreign body in the right mainstem bronchus

stridor or respiratory distress. Endoscopic evaluation is essential for diagnosis. Further imaging with cross-sectional techniques is very helpful to evaluate the distal tracheobronchial tree and detect any concurrent anomalous cardiovascular anatomy, as these may often be seen in association. Symptoms may change as the child grows and respiratory and energy demands increase. Management is tailored to the severity of symptoms and may include nonoperative or expectant management versus open surgery. Slide tracheoplasty has become the favored open surgical

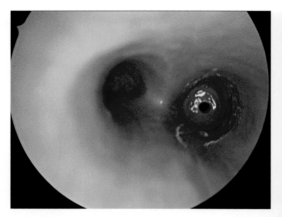

Fig. 4.41 Right mainstem bronchus foreign body (bead)

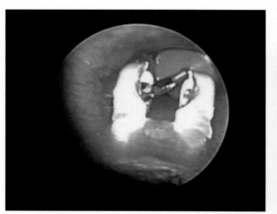

Fig. 4.42 Right mainstem bronchus; thumbtack being removed with optical foreign body forceps

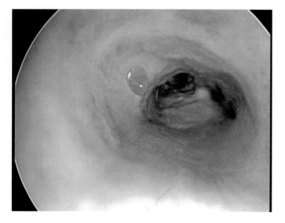

Fig. 4.43 Tracheal stenosis

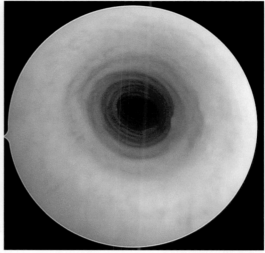

Fig. 4.44 Complete tracheal rings

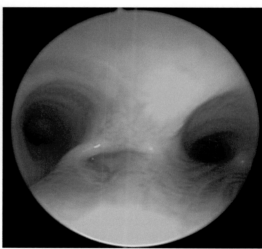

Fig. 4.45 Tracheoesophageal fistula status after repair with blind-ended tracheal pouch

approach [64, 65]. Other operative techniques have been described for long-segment tracheal stenosis, with repair of distal tracheal stenosis often requiring cardiopulmonary bypass [66–68].

Tracheoesophageal Fistula

Tracheoesophageal fistulas are often symptomatic and repaired early in life (Fig. 4.45). Infants who develop feeding issues or respiratory symptoms

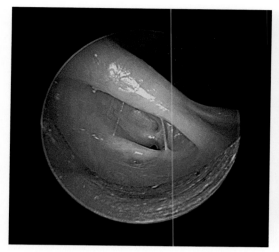

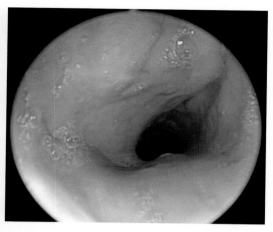

Fig. 4.48 A-frame tracheal stenosis, post-tracheostomy decannulation

Fig. 4.46 Open H-type distal tracheoesophageal fistula

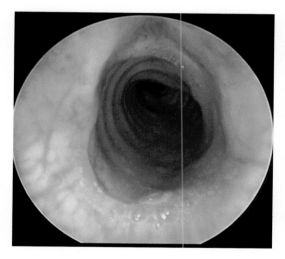

Fig. 4.47 A-frame tracheal stenosis, post-tracheostomy decannulation

after repair of a tracheoesophageal fistula should be investigated urgently with cineradiography and/or endoscopy. If diagnosis of a recurrent fistula is encountered, operative repair should be undertaken. Recurrence is often difficult to manage because revision open surgery is fraught with substantial rates of morbidity, mortality, and further recurrence. Endoscopic repair has been more recently described to manage select children with this problem. Endoscopic diathermy de-epithelialization of the fistula tract

with application of fibrin glue may be successful with minimal morbidity. Congenital H-type fistulas may also be responsive to this management technique (Fig 4.46) [69–72].

A-Frame Tracheal Stenosis

Post-tracheostomy decannulation may be complicated by tracheal stenosis at the site of the tracheostomy (Figs. 4.47 and 4.48). Symptomatic children may require recannulation of the tracheostomy site. Repair of the post-tracheotomy, acquired tracheal stenosis may be successful with anterior cartilage tracheoplasty or cervical slide tracheoplasty [73].

Tracheostomy-Associated Suprastomal Granuloma

Suprastomal granulomas are one of the most common sequelae of long-standing tracheostomies in infants and children. Practice patterns vary widely among pediatric otolaryngologists for surveillance bronchoscopy and management of suprastomal granulomas in children [74]. Often, these lesions are addressed around the time that decannulation is entertained. Open and endoscopic techniques have been described for

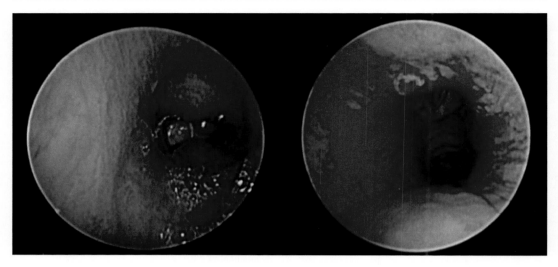

Fig. 4.49 Tracheostomy-associated suprastomal granuloma before (*left*) and after (*right*) removal

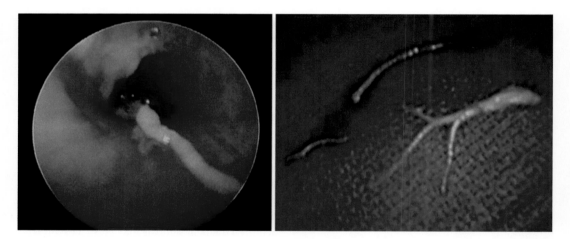

Fig. 4.50 Plastic bronchitis, arborizing casts

management (Fig. 4.49) [75–77]. When identified during interval or surveillance bronchoscopy, excision of nonobstructing granulomas may not be helpful, as recurrence is common [78].

Plastic Bronchitis

Plastic bronchitis in children is characterized by thick, inspissated, mucoid secretions that form arborized casts obstructing the tracheobronchial tree (Fig. 4.50). A high degree of suspicion is necessary to make the diagnosis and should be entertained in the child with respiratory distress that is refractory to standard medical therapy. Two clinical scenarios that may increase the risk of this pathology include asthma exacerbations and status after cardiovascular surgery. Rigid and/or flexible bronchoscopy with aggressive pulmonary toilet and hygiene plays an essential role in management [79–82].

References

1. Garritano FG, Carr MM. Characteristics of patients undergoing supraglottoplasty for laryngomalacia. Int J Pediatr Otorhinolaryngol. 2014;78:1095–100.

2. Dobbie AM, White DR. Laryngomalacia. Pediatr Clin North Am. 2013;60:893–902.

3. Ayari S, Aubertin G, Girschig H, Van Den Abbeele T, Mondain M. Pathophysiology and diagnostic approach to laryngomalacia in infants. Eur Ann Otorhinolaryngol Head Neck Dis. 2012;129:257–63.

4. Kishimoto Y, Hirano S, Kato N, Suehiro A, Kanemaru S, Ito J. Endoscopic KTP laser photocoagulation therapy for pharyngolaryngeal venous malformations in adults. Ann Otol Rhinol Laryngol. 2008;117:881–5.

5. Nouraei SA, Sandhu GS. Treatment of airway compromise due to laryngeal venous malformations: our experience of four patients. Clin Otolaryngol. 2013; 38:174–7.

6. Menon UK, Deepthi NV, Menon IR. Suprahyoid pharyngotomy for excision of laryngeal venous malformation. Ear Nose Throat J. 2012;91:E4–7.

7. Berg EE, Sobol SE, Jacobs I. Laryngeal obstruction by cervical and endolaryngeal lymphatic malformations in children: proposed staging system and review of treatment. Ann Otol Rhinol Laryngol. 2013;122:575–81.

8. Bajaj Y, Hewitt R, Ifeacho S, Hartley BE. Surgical excision as primary treatment modality for extensive cervicofacial lymphatic malformations in children. Int J Pediatr Otorhinolaryngol. 2011;75:673–7.

9. Adams MT, Saltzman B, Perkins JA. Head and neck lymphatic malformation treatment: a systematic review. Otolaryngol Head Neck Surg. 2012;147: 627–39.

10. Hermansen MN, Schmidt JH, Krug AH, Larsen K, Kristensen S. Low incidence of children with acute epiglottis after introduction of vaccination. Dan Med J. 2014;61:A4788.

11. Tibballs J, Watson T. Symptoms and signs differentiating croup and epiglottitis. J Paediatr Child Health. 2011;47:77–82.

12. Guardiani E, Bliss M, Harley E. Supraglottitis in the era following widespread immunization against Haemophilus influenzae type B: evolving principles in diagnosis and management. Laryngoscope. 2010;120:2183–8.

13. Prowse S, Knight L. Congenital cysts of the infant larynx. Int J Pediatr Otorhinolaryngol. 2012;76:708–11.

14. Gonik N, Smith LP. Radiofrequency ablation of pediatric vallecular cysts. Int J Pediatr Otorhinolaryngol. 2012;76:1819–22.

15. Tsai YT, Lee LA, Fang TJ, Li HY. Treatment of vallecular cysts in infants with and without coexisting laryngomalacia using endoscopic laser marsupialization: fifteen-year experience at a single-center. Int J Pediatr Otorhinolaryngol. 2013;77:424–8.

16. Hartnick CJ, Rehbar R, Prasad V. Development and maturation of the pediatric human vocal fold lamina propria. Laryngoscope. 2005;115:4–15.

17. Ambrosio A, Magit A. Respiratory distress of the newborn: congenital laryngeal atresia. Int J Pediatr Otorhinolaryngol. 2012;76:1685–7.

18. Saadai P, Jelin EB, Nijagal A, Schecter SC, Hirose S, MacKenzie TC, et al. Long-term outcomes after fetal therapy for congenital high airway obstructive syndrome. J Pediatr Surg. 2012;47:1095–100.

19. Hamid-Sowinska A, Ropacka-Lesiak M, Breborowicz GH. Congenital high airway obstruction syndrome. Neuro Endocrinol Lett. 2011;32:623–6.

20. de Groot-van der Mooren MD, Haak MC, Lakeman P, Cohen-Overbeek TE, van der Voorn JP, Bretschneider JH, et al. Tracheal agenesis: approach towards this severe diagnosis. Case report and review of the literature. Eur J Pediatr. 2012;171:425–31.

21. Garg MK. Case report: antenatal diagnosis of congenital high airway obstruction syndrome—laryngeal atresia. Indian J Radiol Imaging. 2008;18:350–1.

22. Paniello RC, Desai SC, Allen CT, Khosla SM. Endoscopic keel placement to treat and prevent anterior glottic webs. Ann Otol Rhinol Laryngol. 2013;122:672–8.

23. Edwards J, Tanna N, Bielamowicz SA. Endoscopic lysis of anterior glottic webs and silicone keel placement. Ann Otol Rhinol Laryngol. 2007;116:211–6.

24. Su CY, Alswiahb JN, Hwang CF, Hsu CM, Wu PY, Huang HH. Endoscopic laser anterior commissurotomy for anterior glottic web: one-stage procedure. Ann Otol Rhinol Laryngol. 2010;119:297–303.

25. Amir M, Youssef T. Congenital glottic web: management and anatomical observation. Clin Respir J. 2010;4:202–7.

26. Sztano B, Torkos A, Rovo L. The combined endoscopic management of congenital laryngeal web. Int J Pediatr Otorhinolaryngol. 2010;74:212–5.

27. Hardingham M, Walsh-Waring GP. The treatment of a congenital laryngeal web. J Laryngol Otol. 1975; 89:273–9.

28. Cheng AT, Beckenham EJ. Congenital anterior glottic webs with subglottic stenosis: surgery using perichondrial keels. Int J Pediatr Otorhinolaryngol. 2009; 73:945–9.

29. Wiatrak BJ, Wiatrak DW, Broker TR, Lewis L. Recurrent respiratory papillomatosis: a longitudinal study comparing severity associated with human papilloma viral types 6 and 11 and other risk factors in a large pediatric population. Laryngoscope. 2004; 114(11 Pt 2 Suppl 104):1–23.

30. Heller AJ, Wohl DL. Vocal fold granuloma induced by rigid bronchoscopy. Ear Nose Throat J. 1999;78(3): 176–8. 180.

31. Kelly SM, April MM, Tunkel DE. Obstructing laryngeal granuloma after brief endotracheal intubation in neonates. Otolaryngol Head Neck Surg. 1996; 115(1):138–40.

32. Caroll LM, Mudd P, Zur KB. Severity of voice handicap in children diagnosed with elevated lesions. Otolaryngol Head Neck Surg. 2013; 149(4):628–32.

33. Wentzel JL, Ahmad SM, Discolo CM, Gillespie MB, Dobbie AM, White DR. Balloon laryngoplasty for pediatric laryngeal stenosis: case series and systematic review. Laryngoscope. 2014;124:1707–12.

34. Lang M, Brietzke SE. A systematic review and meta-analysis of endoscopic balloon dilation of pediatric

subglottic stenosis. Otolaryngol Head Neck Surg. 2014;150:174–9.
35. Bajaj Y, Cochrane LA, Jephson CG, et al. Laryngotracheal reconstruction and cricotracheal resection in children: recent experience at Great Ormond Street Hospital. Int J Pediatr Otorhinolaryngol. 2012;76:507–11.
36. Boardman SJ, Albert DM. Single-stage and multi-stage pediatric laryngotracheal reconstruction. Otolaryngol Clin North Am. 2008;41:947–58. ix.
37. Bailey M, Hoeve H, Monnier P. Paediatric laryngotracheal stenosis: a consensus paper from three European centres. Eur Arch Otorhinolaryngol. 2003;260:118–23.
38. Gustafson LM, Hartley BE, Liu JH, et al. Single-stage laryngotracheal reconstruction in children: a review of 200 cases. Otolaryngol Head Neck Surg. 2000;123:430–4.
39. Cotton RT. Management of subglottic stenosis. Otolaryngol Clin North Am. 2000;33:111–30.
40. Richardson MA, Winford TW, Norris BK, Reed JM. Management of pediatric subglottic cysts using the Bugbee fulgurating electrode. JAMA Otolaryngol Head Neck Surg. 2014;140:164–8.
41. Ransom ER, Antunes MB, Smith LP, Jacobs IN. Microdebrider resection of acquired subglottic cysts: case series and review of the literature. Int J Pediatr Otorhinolaryngol. 2009;73:1833–6.
42. Aksoy EA, Elsurer C, Serin GM, Unal OF. Evaluation of pediatric subglottic cysts. Int J Pediatr Otorhinolaryngol. 2012;76:240–3.
43. Lim J, Hellier W, Harcourt J, Leighton S, Albert D. Subglottic cysts: the Great Ormond Street experience. Int J Pediatr Otorhinolaryngol. 2003;67:461–5.
44. Denoyelle F, Leboulanger N, Enjolras O, Harris R, Roger G, Garabedian EN. Role of propranolol in the therapeutic strategy of infantile laryngotracheal hemangioma. Int J Pediatr Otorhinolaryngol. 2009;73: 1168–72.
45. Jephson CG, Manunza F, Syed S, Mills NA, Harper J, Hartley BE. Successful treatment of isolated subglottic haemangioma with propranolol alone. Int J Pediatr Otorhinolaryngol. 2009;73:1821–3.
46. Bajaj Y, Kapoor K, Ifeacho S, Jephson CG, Albert DM, Harper JI, et al. Great Ormond Street Hospital treatment guidelines for use of propranolol in infantile isolated subglottic haemangioma. J Laryngol Otol. 2013;127:295–8.
47. Javia LR, Zur KB, Jacobs IN. Evolving treatments in the management of laryngotracheal hemangiomas: will propranolol supplant steroids and surgery? Int J Pediatr Otorhinolaryngol. 2011;75:1450–4.
48. Lin CD, Cheng YK, Chang JS, Lin HJ, Su BH, Tsai MH. Endoscopic survey of post-extubation stridor in children. Acta Paediatr Taiwan. 2002;43(2):91–5.
49. Goldhagen JL. Croup: pathogenesis and management. J Emerg Med. 1983;1(1):3–11.
50. Mandal A, Kabra SK, Lodha R. Upper airway obstruction in children. Indian J Pediatr. 2015;82(8):737–44.
51. Benjamin B. Airway management in acute infectious croup syndromes. Indian J Otolaryngol Head Neck Surg. 1997;49(3):269–73.
52. Horn DL, DeMarre K, Parikh SR. Interarytenoid sodium carboxymethylcellulose gel injection for management of pediatric aspiration. Ann Otol Rhinol Laryngol. 2014;123:852–8.
53. Cohen MS, Zhuang L, Simons JP, Chi DH, Maguire RC, Mehta DK. Injection laryngoplasty for type 1 laryngeal cleft in children. Otolaryngol Head Neck Surg. 2011;144:789–93.
54. Hoff SR, Koltai PJ. The "postcricoid cushion": observations on the vascular anatomy of the posterior cricoid region. Arch Otolaryngol Head Neck Surg. 2012;138:562–71.
55. Nicoucar K, Giger R, Pope Jr HG, Jaecklin T, Dulguerov P. Management of congenital fourth branchial arch anomalies: a review and analysis of published cases. J Pediatr Surg. 2009;44:1432–9.
56. Shrime M, Kacker A, Bent J, Ward RF. Fourth branchial complex anomalies: a case series. Int J Pediatr Otorhinolaryngol. 2003;67:1227–33.
57. Nicollas R, Ducroz V, Garabedian EN, Triglia JM. Fourth branchial pouch anomalies: a study of six cases and review of the literature. Int J Pediatr Otorhinolaryngol. 1998;44:5–10.
58. Nicoucar K, Giger R, Jaecklin T, Pope Jr HG, Dulguerov P. Management of congenital third branchial arch anomalies: a systematic review. Otolaryngol Head Neck Surg. 2010;142:21–8. e22.
59. Sidell DR, Kim IA, Coker TR, Moreno C, Shapiro NL. Food choking hazards in children. Int J Pediatr Otorhinolaryngol. 2013;77:1940–6.
60. Cutrone C, Pedruzzi B, Tava G, Emanuelli E, Barion U, Fischetto D, et al. The complimentary role of diagnostic and therapeutic endoscopy in foreign body aspiration in children. Int J Pediatr Otorhinolaryngol. 2011;75:1481–5.
61. Zur KB, Litman RS. Pediatric airway foreign body retrieval: surgical and anesthetic perspectives. Paediatr Anaesth. 2009;19 Suppl 1:109–17.
62. Zerella JT, Dimler M, McGill LC, Pippus KJ. Foreign body aspiration in children: value of radiography and complications of bronchoscopy. J Pediatr Surg. 1998;33:1651–4.
63. Erikci V, Karacay S, Arikan A. Foreign body aspiration: a four-years experience. Ulus Travma Acil Cerrahi Derg. 2003;9:45–9.
64. Rutter MJ, Willging JP, Cotton RT. Nonoperative management of complete tracheal rings. Arch Otolaryngol Head Neck Surg. 2004;130:450–2.
65. Rutter MJ, Cotton RT, Azizkhan RG, Manning PB. Slide tracheoplasty for the management of complete tracheal rings. J Pediatr Surg. 2003;38:928–34.
66. Valencia D, Overman D, Tibesar R, Lander T, Moga F, Sidman J. Surgical management of distal tracheal stenosis in children. Laryngoscope. 2011;121:2665–71.
67. Wijeweera O, Ng SB. Retrospective review of tracheoplasty for congenital tracheal stenosis. Singapore Med J. 2011;52:726–9.

68. Backer CL, Mavroudis C, Holinger LD. Repair of congenital tracheal stenosis. Semin Thorac Cardiovasc Surg Pediatr Card Surg Annu. 2002;5:173–86.

69. Richter GT, Ryckman F, Brown RL, Rutter MJ. Endoscopic management of recurrent tracheo-esophageal fistula. J Pediatr Surg. 2008;43:238–45.

70. Tzifa KT, Maxwell EL, Chait P, James AL, Forte V, Ein SH, et al. Endoscopic treatment of congenital H-type and recurrent tracheoesophageal fistula with electrocautery and histoacryl glue. Int J Pediatr Otorhinolaryngol. 2006;70:925–30.

71. Lopes MF, Pires J, Nogueria Brandao A, Reis A, Morais Leitao L. Endoscopic obliteration of a recurrent tracheoesophageal fistula with enbucrilate and polidocanol in a child. Surg Endosc. 2003;17:657.

72. Ghandour KE, Spitz L, Brereton RJ, Kiely EM. Recurrent tracheo-oesophageal fistula: experience with 24 patients. J Paediatr Child Health. 1990;26:89–91.

73. de Alarcon A, Rutter MJ. Cervical slide tracheoplasty. Arch Otolaryngol Head Neck Surg. 2012;138:812–6.

74. Kraft S, Patel S, Sykes K, Nicklaus P, Gratny L, Wei JL. Practice patterns after tracheotomy in infants younger than 2 years. Arch Otolaryngol Head Neck Surg. 2011;137:670–4.

75. Gallagher TQ, Hartnick CJ. Suprastomal granuloma. Adv Otorhinolaryngol. 2012;73:63–5.

76. Kitsko DJ, Chi DH. Coblation removal of large suprastomal tracheal granulomas. Laryngoscope. 2009;119:387–9.

77. Gupta A, Cotton RT, Rutter MJ. Pediatric suprastomal granuloma: management and treatment. Otolaryngol Head Neck Surg. 2004;131:21–5.

78. Rosenfeld RM, Stool SE. Should granulomas be excised in children with long-term tracheotomy? Arch Otolaryngol Head Neck Surg. 1992;118:1323–7.

79. Goldberg DJ, Dodds K, Rychik J. Rare problems associated with the Fontan circulation. Cardiol Young. 2010;20 Suppl 3:113–9.

80. Healy F, Hanna BD, Zinman R. Pulmonary complications of congenital heart disease. Paediatr Respir Rev. 2012;13:10–5.

81. Cairns-Bazarian AM, Conway Jr EE, Yankelowitz S. Plastic bronchitis: an unusual cause of respiratory distress in children. Pediatr Emerg Care. 1992;8:335–7.

82. Noizet O, Leclerc F, Leteurtre S, Brichet A, Pouessel G, Dorkenoo A, et al. Plastic bronchitis mimicking foreign body aspiration that needs a specific diagnostic procedure. Intensive Care Med. 2003;29:329–31.

Index

© Springer International Publishing Switzerland 2016
J. Cheng, J.P. Bent (eds.), *Endoscopic Atlas of Pediatric Otolaryngology*,
DOI 10.1007/978-3-319-29471-1

Printed in the United States
By Bookmasters